Cure Craft

by the same author

Homoeopathy for the Third Age
Homoeopathy: Heart & Soul

Dr Keith M. Souter
DSc, MB, ChB, MRCGP, MHMA

Cure Craft

Traditional Folk Remedies
and Treatment from Antiquity
to the present day

Index compiled
by Lyn Greenwood

Saffron Walden
The C.W. Daniel Company Limited

First published in Great Britain by
The C.W. Daniel Company Limited
1 Church Path, Saffron Walden
Essex, CB10 1JP, England

ISBN 0 85207 282 1

This book is not intended to replace orthodox medical care or
advice. It has been written primarily for interest and in order
to provide a record of oral Folk Medicine. Whilst every care
has been taken to exclude herbs which could be dangerous,
the author and publisher cannot accept any responsibility
for any situation or problem which could arise from
experimentation with any of these remedies. If in doubt
about a medical problem, the individual should consult
their professional health advisor.

This book is printed on part-recycled paper

Designed and produced by Book Production Consultants
Typeset by Cambridge Photosetting Services
Printed by St Edmundsbury Press, Suffolk

For my mother, Mollie McDonald Souter, who has taught me
so much about Scottish Folk Medicine throughout my life.
With grateful thanks and love.

Contents

Acknowledgements

I wish to express my gratitude to several people who have helped me greatly in the production of this book.

First of all I would like to say a special thanks to the late John Bunnell, my good and sadly missed friend, who helped me to see that there was a need to record the oral tradition of Folk Medicine.

I thank Ian Miller of the C.W. Daniel Co Ltd, for his discernment, encouragement, patience, and absolutely unique sense of humour. In the same breath I thank Jane Miller, whose immensely gifted powers of persuasion have resulted in my previous books being published abroad. I feel priviledged, and a little humbled, to have my books published on the same list as some of the truly great names in Natural Medicine.

As ever, I thank Rachel, Katherine, Ruth and Andrew for their consideration when I was busy writing, instead of spending time with them.

Thanks must go to Derrick Biggart who almost literally dragged me screaming into the twentieth century. Without his help I would never have mastered the technology which has enabled me to write and illustrate this book without actually ever putting pen to paper.

Finally, a big thanks to all my other relatives, patients and colleagues who have freely informed me about Folk remedies that they have used or been told about at some stage in their lives. Indeed, to all the people who have kept the oral tradition of Medicine alive over many centuries, I thank you.

Introduction

*"But know also, man has an inborn
craving for medicine ... the desire to
take medicine is one feature which
distinguishes man the animal, from
his fellow creatures."*

Sir William Osler, 1894

Folk Medicine is a blanket description for a whole host of remedies, treatments and practices which have been, or are still being used by people as a means of self-help. Whereas we associate the term 'Traditional' with complete medical systems such as Acupuncture, Chinese Herbal Medicine and Indian Unani and Ayurvedic Medicine, the concept of Folk Medicine is much broader. It is an accumulate of medical practices which crosses geographical borders, and extends from the early days of history until the present time. It has no central theme, no written canon and no officially recognised practitioners. Nevertheless, throughout the world it is the form of medicine which is used by over seventy-five per cent of the population.

In the UK for example, when someone feels ill, only one per cent of the population will attend a hospital, about twenty-five per cent will attend some sort of practitioner (a GP or complementary medicine professional) and the rest will resort to some form of self-treatment.

In the rural areas of less developed Third World countries, many people may never see a trained health worker such as a doctor, nurse or midwife. In such cases, their only alternative might be to use some form of Folk Medicine. Indeed, two thirds of the world's babies are brought into the world by non-qualified Folk Medicine attendants.

With the development of modern Medicine and the establishment of health care systems like the National Health Service, much of our traditional Folk Medicine has started to disappear. This could be a tragedy, because there is undoubtedly much wisdom in these truly traditional practices. Many accepted modern treatments are based on the lore of bygone days and there is undoubtedly more to be learned. Unless we keep the subject alive we may well lose that wisdom forever.

Within this book you will find magical remedies, love potions and charms, herbal and traditional remedies, some of them dating back to Antiquity. For easy reading I have divided the book into two sections. Part one covers the principles by which Folk Medicines and remedies were and are derived. Part two takes the form of an A-Z index covering common symptoms and conditions and the remedies which have or are still being used in Folk Medicine.

The amazing thing about Folk Medicine is that it has survived across the centuries mainly as a result of oral tradition. Ironically, as technology and science improve communications to turn our world into a global village, they are destroying our ability to actually communicate the old ways. The aim of this book is to at least keep the old knowledge alive for our children and our children's children.

KEITH SOUTER

SECTION ONE

1 What is Folk Medicine?

2 Magic and Medicine

3 Medical Divination

4 Follow the signs

5 Vital Fluids and Vital Herbs

6 Airs, Waters and Places

7 Fertility Rites and Love Charms

8 Natural Tonics

9 The Monk, The Blacksmith and the Farmer's Wife

Chapter One

What is Folk Medicine?

For every ill beneath the sun
There is some remedy or none;
If there be one, resolve to find it;
If not, submit, and never mind it.

Old English Folk Maxim

You may wonder why a scientifically trained doctor should become involved in the study of Folk Medicine. Permit me to explain.

Like just about every child in the British Isles, at about the age of four I was taught that dock leaves are good for nettle stings. As a teenager, coming from the family that I did (a Scottish family with its roots firmly in the Highlands) I also knew that a well worn sock wrapped round the neck and left overnight was supposed to be good for curing sores throats, and that there were at least five ways of curing warts. My knowledge of omens was fair, I had some idea of weather-lore and I had been taught to dowse by my grandfather.

None of this, of course, was to be of the remotest use to me when I entered medical school. Indeed, after several years of hard medical science I became a staunch rationalist. By the time I graduated, I had written all of my folklore knowledge off as nonsense.

Some years later while working in general practice I had a learning experience which re-kindled my interest in Folk Medicine. For several weeks I had been vainly struggling to help a patient with a back problem. I had tried all of the accepted conventional medical treatments, but without any success whatsoever. I was surprised, therefore, to see him fairly march into my consulting-room one morning. He grinned broadly as he stood to attention by the desk, then suddenly jack-knifed forward to touch his toes. Before I could congratulate him he whipped a filthy-looking bottle out of his pocket, uncorked it and wafted it under my nose.

It smelled awful.

'Deldoc!' he announced. 'Friend of mine treats his animals with it. Works a treat.'

It was some time later that I discovered what it was. Correctly, it was called *Opodeldoc*, a camphorated soap liniment which had been devised by Paracelsus in the early sixteenth century.

A few weeks after this I was fortunate enough to meet my patient's farmer friend. He was not exactly impressed by the medical profession. Indifferent would be a fair description. He'd never had need of us, you see. He applied natural remedies to himself and his family, just as he did to his livestock. His 'learning' had been passed on to him by his parents.

I asked him what he used if Deldoc failed.

'Hurtication,' he replied. Then he outlined his method of harvesting fresh nettles and flailing the painful part and surrounding area. One could see why it was called that. It would be bound to hurt.

After some thought, however, it dawned on me that perhaps this remedy might also have undergone a name change over the years. And so it seemed. For hurtication, read *Urtication*.

Urtication, from the Latin *urtica* for nettle, is a technique of considerable antiquity. In a form it was used by the Romans for the treatment of rheumatic and circulatory disorders, and in medieval times it was used to treat bed-wetting children.

The more remedies that my new acquaintance came out with, the more fascinated I became. It awakened my dormant interest in Folk Medicine and I was spurred on to research the methods he outlined. Over the years I discovered remedies, charms, talismans and amulets. I found that some had underlying theories which indicated foreign origins, archaic philosophies and sometimes linked up with past documented medical practice. To my utter fascination, I discovered that Folk Medicine was a living phenomenon, kept going through oral tradition. Admittedly it has been on the decline since the Great War, yet there are still many people out there keeping the old traditions alive. And in doing so they are still practising methods which have in some cases come down to us from the dawn of mankind.

'Superstition!' 'Gypsy cures!' 'Old wive's tales!'

These are some of the derogatory labels which are often hurled at the practices which make up the rich tapestry of Folk Medicine. Admittedly, all three labels have some truth attached to them, yet that truth is not nearly so disparaging as the way it is intended.

Folk Medicine is an amalgamation of different practices which over the centuries filtered into a pool of oral tradition. Those practices reflect the magical beliefs, or superstitions which are almost innate in human beings, whether they admit it or not. Similarly many of them have 'come from afar', having been spread across the world by Gypsies and travellers of all sorts. And finally, they have been kept alive by the 'old wives,' the wise women of local communities.

Folk Medicine in the British Isles can trace its roots to Ancient Egypt, Classical Greece, Rome, Arabia, the Vikings and the Normans. Some practices mirror medical traditions of the far East and of the Americas.

Essentially, Folk Medicine illustrates the flow of ideas across the world. Practices which were once part of the accepted core of medical knowledge passed into the community and were by and large kept alive through oral tradition.

Magic, Religion and Science

It is said that Medicine has evolved through the phases of magic, religion and science. From the days of prehistory to the rise of the cradle lands of civilisation, magical forces would have been thought responsible for every phenomenon upon the Earth. Illness in those far off days was thought to be due to possession by demons. Treatments were barbaric and brutal. Archaeological finds around the world attest to the commonly performed procedure of trephination, the boring of a hole in the skull in order to let out the demon.

Over the centuries magico-medical rituals would have developed and been absorbed into the core of wisdom of the rising priestly classes. Evidence from Ancient Egypt, Babylon and Ancient China all show this phase of medical evolution. Deities were worshipped as the patrons of healing, and medical priesthoods developed.

Slowly, as the ancient empires filtered outwards, their influence being carried on by succeeding cultures, the hold of religion would have given way to the development of science. It is the Greeks that we immediately think of in this context, for they developed the arts of mathematics, logic and medicine.

The phases of magic, religion and science are inextricably bound up with medicine. Although we think that we have entered the truly scientific age, yet are we still shackled to our innate need to hold to a belief system. To the scientist the belief may be in science, to the theologian it is belief in the spirit, and to the atheist it is belief in non-belief. These are our rational beliefs. For most of us, there is a deeper, almost unconscious belief which is particularly hard to relinquish. It is the belief in magic.

Even though one consciously rejects it, there still remains the deep-rooted idea that perhaps there are such powers. For example, there is hardly a person who does not have some little superstition, some little charm, ritual or mental affirmation in particular circumstances. And whether they like it or not, that means that they have a belief in magic. That belief is one of the factors which has kept the oral tradition of Folk Medicine alive.

As suggested above, Folk Medicine is an amalgamation of different practices which have filtered over the centuries into a pool of oral tradition. One can think of the phases of magic, religion and science as the clouds of thought which have shed their load upon the mountain of human understanding. As they have fallen, their waters have caused a river to stream down the mountain. This is the surface layer of accepted or mainstream Medicine (Figure 1). But as ideas have changed, so the influences have seeped through the mountain to accumulate in a great un-conscious, subterranean pool of knowledge. At times this great

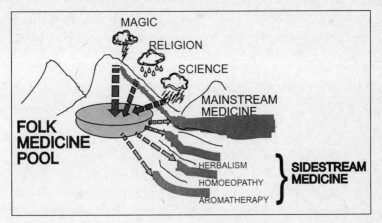

Figure 1

gathering pool of Folk Medicine has contributed to the river of mainstream Medicine, such as when drugs like aspirin, digoxin and some antibiotics have been discovered from observations of Folk practice. Similarly, other channels have burst through as springs, to form parallel streams to that of Medicine. We have seen this in the development of various complementary therapies, again after observation of Folk practice. We shall touch upon this again later in the book.

The flow of ideas

There are some remarkable similarities between the Folk Medicine practices of countries across the globe. The practices in the British Isles, for example, seem to have roots which extend back to Ancient Egypt, Arabia, the Aegean Isles of Classical Greece, Rome, the Celts and the Normans.

Folk Medicine illustrates the flow of ideas across the world. However, because Folk Medicine is essentially an oral tradition, the origin of remedies, charms and treatments is not always clear. Three factors are worth considering. Firstly, the spread of language. Secondly, the spread of religion. Finally, the spread of different philosophies.

It is estimated that there are some 4,000 to 5,000 distinct

languages in the world. All of these can be fitted into about six language families. In other words, they can be traced back to one of the common ancestor languages. These are:–

Indo-European, which includes many of the world's classical languages, including Latin, Greek, and many of the European, Northern Indian and Latin American languages.

Hamito-Semitic, which has two main branches. The Hamitic group are mainly found in the North of Africa and include Ancient Egyptian, Coptic and Berber. The Semitic group had their origin in Mesopotamia, Syria, Palestine and Arabia. These include Arabic, Hebrew, Syriac and Aramaic.

Finno-Ugric, which includes some 20 Scandinavian languages from Norway in the West to Siberia in the East.

Sino-Tibetan, which cover most of the languages of South-east Asia, including Chinese, Burmese, and Tai.

Malayo-Polynesian, which cover the languages of Malaysia, Indonesia, Polynesia, including Malay and Maori.

Uto-Aztecan, which include many of the languages of the Americas.

The significance of the language families is that although language spreads (Figure 2), it remains concentrated in the geographical areas in which it thrived most. Clearly, this would be likely to include its ancestral origin as well as the parts of the world to which people moved in substantial numbers. And this would seem to have followed the expansion of empires.

For example, the Indo-European family includes the languages of Latin, Greek, Italian, Spanish, French, English, and Gaelic. They cover the geographical areas which were settled by the Greek and Roman Empires, by the Celts, the Angles, Saxons and Normans. Throughout this whole great area, the cultures are generally very similar.

By culture, I refer to the shared customs, traditions and beliefs

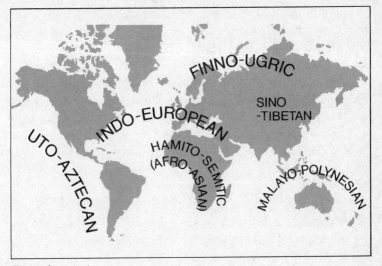

Figure 2

of the people. This includes their thoughts about illness, remedies and treatments. In other words, it includes the Folk Medicine of the population. It is particularly interesting to note the many instances of similar Folk remedies in cultures which are geographically very distant from one another. Obvious examples are the similarities between parts of Europe and Latin America.

Religion is another marker for the flow of thought. As a religious practice spreads across the world it seems to be followed by aspects of the culture in which that religion arose. In many such cases the religious practice has not stood the test of time, but has died out. Sometimes, however, aspects of it persist as they have filtered into the realm of folklore. Again, there are many examples of medical practices from ancient times which seem to have fallen into the knowledge pool of Folk Medicine. The use of scarabs or beetles in different ways, for example, indicates an Ancient Egyptian pedigree. Similarly, the recurring symbol of the crescent moon in superstition and talismanic magic refers back to the spread of the cult of the Egyptian goddess Isis.

Finally, as different philosophical systems have developed, the whole structure of knowledge has changed. Ideas which were once part of established thought were discarded. Science has repeatedly caused this over the centuries and resulted in previously established practices being discredited and jettisoned. Yet this very act of jettisoning does not mean that the ideas have been abandoned and lost forever. Indeed, to take herbalism as an example, the underlying humoral theories were supposedly disproved during the seventeenth and eighteenth centuries, yet it continued to be practised as an integral part of Folk Medicine. And it was from there that it was subsequently rescued and 're-discovered' to become one of today's major Complementary Medicines.

'Epochs of change'

The history of Medicine is a fascinating study, yet for our purposes we can look at particular epochs which resulted in the spread and movement of medical knowledge.

FROM SHAMAN TO PRIEST

Illness is an inevitable accompaniment of life. The earliest humans, so vulnerable to a huge range of illness, accidents and early death, true to their hunting way of existence sought to placate their gods and to search for cures. As the early tribal societies developed it is probable that within the tribe a single individual would accumulate the knowledge about healing. It would be he or she who would communicate with the gods and seek out the animals and herbs needed for ceremonies and medicines. This individual, the wise person, the shaman, the witch-doctor, would cater for the well-being of the other members.

So important would this knowledge be, that the shaman would teach an apprentice. The shaman's untimely death would have been considered a tragedy, since the knowledge would be lost forever. And in those early days the only way that the knowledge could be passed on was through oral tradition.

With the development of actual societies the role of the shaman would probably become more formalised and develop into a sort of priesthood. Indeed, the evidence from the early civilisations shows that the first physicians belonged to the priest classes, an almost inevitable situation considering that illness was thought to have a supernatural basis.

THE CRADLE LANDS OF CIVILISATION

The first recorded guidelines for physicians dates back to Babylon around the year 1900 BC, when the Code of King Hammurabi was inscribed. We know that three types of Mesopotamian priests were involved in medicine. First there was the *baru,* who used divination to diagnose and prognosticate about illnesses and other disasters. The *ashipu* was called upon to exorcise demons causing illness. And finally, the *asu* prepared amulets and talismans, prepared medicines and conducted rituals and operations.

The Ancient Egyptians developed a more 'scientific' form of medicine. Although their civilisation is popularly assumed to have been obsessed with death and the after-life, their knowledge of medicine was appreciable. At the time of writing this book, there are seven known medical papyruses. Of these, the two most illuminating are the Edwin Smith Papyrus from about 1700 BC, which deals with surgery; and the Ebers Papyrus from about 1600 BC, which lists some 700 drugs, charms and incantations.

Very importantly the Ebers papyrus also contains a reference to one of the most significant medical discoveries of all time – the use of the pill as a means of taking medication. This was an incredibly sophisticated idea, since before that time medicines had to be taken in the form of soups, potions and other nauseus concoctions. To be able to take medicines in a solid and transportable form was completely revolutionary.

MEDICINE IN CLASSICAL GREECE

It is to Classical Greece that most people turn their minds, how-ever, when thinking of the birth of Medicine. In particular, to the Island of Cos, the home of the great physician, Hippocrates. Upon this island the cult of Aesculapius, the main Greek god of healing, was practised. In many ways this god was similar to the deified physician and pyramid architect Imhotep of Egypt. Indeed, this influence is quite likely, since early Greek thought was probably influenced by the flow of ideas from two sources. Firstly, into Ionia from Mesopotamia to the North. Secondly, from Egypt and Crete, thence to mainland Greece.

Up until the middle of the fifth century BC, Greek Medicine was essentially an off-shoot of religion. The sick were tended in the temples dedicated to Aesculapius, by the priest-physicians known as the Aesclepiads. There they made sacrifices, prayed and slept after the administration of hypnotic drugs. The interpretation of dreams was considered of crucial importance.

According to the history of Soranus, Hippocrates was born in the year of the 80th Olympiad (about 460 BC) into a family of Aesclepiads. After travelling widely throughout the Aegean he returned to Cos where he taught his system of Medicine. It was his belief that illness was not a result of some supernatural force, but that it was attributable to disorders of the body itself. He recognised that in trying to help the individual the physician had to wait for *Vis Medicatrix Naturae*, the healing power of nature.

The Hippocratic approach rapidly spread throughout the world of Classical Greece. A series of texts known as the Hippocratic Canon have come down to us. Several of the texts are believed to have been written by the great physician himself, although there is now evidence to suggest that the actual Hippocratic Oath was written much later by several authors. Nonetheless, the spirit of the Hippocratic method was to have a profound influence on medical thought until the present day.

The Greek Empire spread over the following years, reaching its zenith under the generalship of Alexander the Great. He extended its dominions across Persia and into India, and across Arabia into Egypt. It was there that the city of Alexandria was founded in 332 BC. Strikingly, since Alexander had been the pupil of Aristotle, a major seat of learning was established there. Its most significant feature was the inclusion of a medical school based upon the Hippocratic method.

THE PTOLEMAIC PERIOD

When Alexander the Great died in 323 BC, the rule of Egypt fell to one of his field commanders who became Ptolemy 1. This was to be the start of a three hundred year dynasty which ended when Cleopatra, the last Ptolemy died after a self-inflicted asp bite.

The significance of the Ptolemaic Period is that there was a fascinating amalgamation of beliefs. Egyptian gods were mixed with Greek deities, and Egyptian and Greek Medicine were cross-fertilised. The perfect conditions were created for the spread of knowledge across the seas. This was to happen as the Roman Empire spread across the world.

MEDICINE IN THE ROMAN EMPIRE

In the first century BC, a Greek physician, Asclepiades of Bithynia attained great fame in Rome, where he founded the *methodical school* of medicine. Unlike Hippocrates he advocated using contraries (or medicines which were opposite to the illness symptoms), as well as generous diets, strenuous exercise and bathing. It is likely that this physician was largely responsible for introducing the Roman ideal of frequent baths, and indirectly responsible for the enthusiasm with which the Romans built baths near medicinal springs and wells.

In the first century AD, a Roman encyclopedist, Cornelius Celsus, wrote *De Medicina*. In these vast volumes he covered the medical theories of the day and outlined the operations which were performed for plastic repair of the nose, cutting for bladder stones, repairing hernias and removing tonsils.

A century later, Claudius Galen, a Greek who was personal physician to the Emperor Marcus Aurelius, took up and developed the humoral theory of Hippocrates. Undoubtedly, he was to be the most influential medical writer for more than a millennium. His theories formed the basis of medical practice throughout most of the civilised world until the sixteenth century. Having said that, they are still used in various medical systems throughout the world. Indeed, in herbal and Folk Medicine the influence can still be seen.

THE PERSECUTION OF THE CHRISTIANS

The persecution of the Christians began with the Romans. However, despite the fact that Christianity survived to become a major religion, persecution of groups within the faith was still common. In 431 AD, Nestorius the Patriarch of Constantinople, and his group of followers declared that the virgin Mary was the mother of Jesus on his human side alone, thereby implying that since she was not the mother of God, Jesus had two personalities. Accordingly, he was denounced as a heretic and banished.

It was ultimately to Persia that the Nestorians fled, where they found asylum under the patronage of King Chosroes. Together with the Jews of Gundishapur they formed a medical school, where they began translating Greek texts into Arabic, Syrian and Hebrew.

MEDICINE TRAVELS EAST AND WEST
In 636 AD, the city of Gundishapur was over-run by the Moslems, who absorbed the medical system into their culture. As a result, the medical system was allowed to develop further. And indeed, in a very recognisable form it is still practiced to this very day.

At this point one should note a dual path in the flow of medical knowledge. On the one hand the medical ideas of Hippocrates and Galen became absorbed into the Islamic faith. On the other, they were preserved within the Christian faith as various monastic orders were established throughout Europe and the British isles. Clearly the different religious influences resulted in differences in interpretation. It is true to say, however, that there was more development in the Arabic world, thanks to the contributions of a number of talented and knowledgeable Arabian physicians.

When the Crusaders fought their way across the Holy Land some centuries later, they were astonished to discover the advanced medicine that was being practised. So much so that when they returned home, they brought back much useful knowledge which would have been amalgamated with the medical practice of the monks.

THE DEVELOPMENT OF THE UNIVERSITIES
The Italian sea-port of Salerno in the eleventh century was a truly cosmopolitan city. Merchants from all over the world congregated there, and travellers of every race were welcome. It had been considered a health resort since the time of the Romans and it was a natural setting for a seat of learning. This it duly became when the first medical school in Europe was established.

Over the years the medical curriculum at Salerno became famous. Arabic translations of the works of the Arabian physicians Avicenna and Rhazes, were translated into Latin alongside the works of the Jewish physician Moses Maimonides and those of Celsus, Galen and Hippocrates. Students flocked from all over Europe and 'Western' medicine was born.

In the twelfth and thirteenth centuries the lead which Salerno had shown was followed when other universities were established at Padua, Bologna, Montpellier and Paris. And true to the tradition of Salerno the Graeco-Arabian system was the basis of their medical training.

THE RENNAISANCE AND THE AGE OF EXPLORATION.

The following centuries are rightly regarded as the Age of Exploration. Between the years 1420 and 1620 European merchant adventurers charted the seas of the world and began the process of trade and colonisation. And just as medical ideas were taken to those distant lands, so it was inevitable that local practices would be observed. In time colonists would explore further into the continents and settlements would be established. As a result, there would be a mixing together of traditional and imported medical systems.

At the same time, just as Art and Science were undergoing momentous changes during the Renaissance, the most basic tenets of Medicine were being challenged. A number of scientific discoveries seemed to disprove the humoral theories of Galen. In 1625, for example, Santorio Santorio, a colleague of Galileo, used an early thermometer to show that people with 'cold' and 'hot' constitutions both had very similar temperatures (see Chapter 5). And three years later in 1628 William Harvey demonstrated the circulation of the blood around the body. By substantiating theory with experimental proof they laid the foundations for the science of physiology.

THE DEVELOPMENT OF SCIENCE

At about the same time Rene Descartes, a mathematician, outlined a new philosophical method. His view of the universe was that it was ordered, mechanistic and therefore predictable. He believed that human beings were basically machines designed by God and which were infused by a 'rational soul.' Also, since he perceived man to be superior to animals, he concluded that animals were no more than sophisticated automatons. Therefore, he considered it legitimate for men to discover the manner in which organs worked by carrying out experimentation on animals.

This philosophy, which came to be called Cartesianism, effectively implied that the mind and body were separate and that they could be compartmentalised. Accordingly, different sciences sprang up to analyse different aspects of man. Anatomists dissected the body and ascertained its structure. Physiologists analysed the functioning of the organs. Pathologists studied the effect of disease upon organs.

This process of reductionism has been the pattern of medical science until this very day.

THE SEARCH FOR THE MAGIC BULLET

As Medicine advanced into the nineteenth and twentieth centuries the search for drugs became all important. Vast numbers of illness-modifying agents have been discovered. Antibiotics, the magic bullets which kill off the life threatening infections of the past; anti-depressants which stave off the horrors of depression; insulin, which has saved so many people from the former fatal condition of Diabetes Mellitis – all of them have improved the quality of life for people today.

THE SEARCH FOR THE ALTERNATIVE

In the late twentieth century with Medicine continuing to make great advances one would have thought that people would be satisfied. The truth is that many people are not. There has been an undoubted reaction to the patriarchal approach of modern Medicine which by and large takes responsibility away from the patient and makes him/her the mere recipient of some treatment or another. There has also grown a deep suspicion about drugs and the side effects that they might bring. This has brought about a tendency for people to search for alternative ways of dealing with their health. As a result, a whole host of Alternative therapies have been developed.

The question is immediately posed – where have these Alternatives come from?

The answer is that they have always been there. They are not new. Most actually cite past practices and past wisdom as the stimulus for their development. Their founding fathers have 'rediscovered' these therapies from that vast pool of Folk Medicine.

Culture and Folk Medicine

As Sir William Osler said, man has an inborn craving to take medicine. Certainly every culture has developed a system of

Medicine. And as the accepted Art or Science of Medicine has developed within that culture, so too has it inevitably added to the pool of Folk Medicine. While it is true that Folk practices can be remarkably similar across the globe, it also has to be noted that there are differences too. These differences arise from variations in the medical beliefs of the people within the different cultures.

The French, for example, recognise the symptom complex of *crise de foie,* which is taken to mean that the liver has been over-worked from too much rich food. The treatment is to cleanse the system with plenty of mineral waters.

The British have a great concern for their bowels and describe the problem of being *costive*. Accordingly, they consume a significantly greater amounts of laxatives than other Europeans. They also talk about having taken cold or contracted a *chill*.

The North Americans talk about having *high blood*, which is not to be confused with having high blood pressure. This symptom complex is thought to come about from having too much blood with resultant congestion of different bodily parts.

In addition, there are many other so-called nervous 'Folk illnesses' which are fairly unique to individual cultures. Thus, Malayans might run *amok*, a type of acute hysterical reaction, associated with aggressive tendencies. In China males may suffer from *koro*, a belief that the penis is shrinking and that when it eventually disappears inside the abdomen, death will follow. In Pakistan men might suffer from *jiryan*, a belief that their sperm is leaking into their urine, resulting in lack of potency and vital energy. Latin Americans experience *susto*, a feeling that the soul is slipping away from the physical body.

Also of note are the different beliefs in the lay mind about the way the body works. The further East one goes, the more people think of the body as a balance. Health is equated with equilibrium. In more Western countries the idea of the body as a piece of sophisticated plumbing becomes more common. The British, as stated earlier, very often become fixated with the notion of constipation, blocked bowels and the consequent absorption of toxins from the blocked bowel motions. The Americans, take the idea of the body as a machine to even greater lengths in their high-tech society. The analogy of the body to a piece of technology with internal parts that can be removed, reworked or replaced is quite in keeping with the emphasis of their ever-increasing high-tech medical system and pace of life. Indeed, in Western societies, the analogy of the mind with a computer is being made more and more frequently. People talk about their health with pseudo-computer jargonese. They talk about software problems, burnout, bad programs and of health crashes.

Folk Medicine today

As I mentioned in the introduction, when people feel ill, even in highly developed countries with extensive health care systems, the majority choose to use self help. In Britain up until the Great World War of 1914–18, Folk Medicine was extensively used in all rural populations. My own grandparents depended upon it and taught their children the use of herbs from the fields and hedgerows of the highlands of Scotland. And this was by no means unusual. Even up until the end of the 1950s people were still relying heavily upon Folk remedies. Then, as transistors revolutionised technology and the world started to become a more 'sophisticated', consumer-orientated place, the lore started to retreat.

Yet even today the lore has not gone. People realise more than ever before that they have the right to choose. They can choose conventional medical help or they can help themselves. The form which this self help takes will depend upon the individual and his or her beliefs; how ill they feel they are; and who they turn to for advice.

The options include a whole range of remedies and treatments. They may choose an over-the-counter (OTC) preparation from a pharmacist. They may purchase a herbal-type remedy from a herbalist or health shop. They may manufacture a remedy in a traditional manner. They may take a 'well-tried' family or domestic remedy. Finally, they may resort to some sort of magical remedy.

Studies have shown that the older the person the sufferer consults, the more likely are they to try a traditional Folk remedy. Grandparents are the most likely to advise one to use such a method. On the other hand, the longer the individual has lived in an urban environment, the greater is the likelihood of them consulting a pharmacist and buying an OTC remedy. Finally, and this may surprise you, the last category of magical remedies, which includes the use of charms, talismans and various forms of healing amounts to as much as ten per cent of Folk Medicine used today.

In essence, Folk Medicine is a rich ground for study. It consists of the traditional beliefs of the indigenous population, modified and extended by the influence of travellers, conquerors, and the spread of religion, philosophy and science. It is an oral tradition which is ever-increasing as it receives and maintains the ancient, the domestic and the anecdotal remedies which filter into it from many sources.

In the next few chapters we shall look at some of those rich sources.

Chapter Two

Magic and Medicine

"Thou shalt on paper write the spell divine
ABRACADABRA called in many a line,
Each under each in even order place,
But the last letter in each line efface,
As by degrees the elements grow few,
Still take away but fix the residue,
Till at the last one letter stands alone,
And the whole dwindles to a tapering cone.
Tie this about the neck with flaxen string,
Mighty the good 'twill to the patient bring,
Its mighty potency shall guard his head
And drive disease and death from his bed"

Severus Sammonicus
Third Century AD

In the last chapter I talked about the three phases through which Medicine evolves. To the modern physician, magic and religion have little place in the day to day practice of his profession. Yet things were not always so.

As I write this chapter I am overlooked by a statuette of Imhotep. He sits, scroll of knowledge upon his lap, atop a plinth in my consulting room. The original statue is in to be found in the British Museum, yet my reproduction still has a certain magical significance for me.

Imhotep lived about 2,600 BC. An undoubted genius, in his lifetime he was a vizier, scribe, poet and physician. History proclaims him to have been the architect of the Step pyramid of King Zoser at Saqqara. That apart, he was deified as a healing divinity alongside the god Thoth. For centuries he was invoked during all sorts of healing rituals and treatments.

For me, it is quite fitting that he overlooks my consulting-room which doubles as a study, since his influence extended from the world of healing to the world of the written word.

The point is that although I do not consciously attribute my statuette of Imhotep with supernatural powers, I do enjoy his presence in the room because it somehow feels right that he should be there. I rationalise it by saying that the statuette symbolises good medical and writing practice. And when you think about it, most people do this. They like to have objects near them which 'symbolise' the activity or occupation they are involved in. It may be a framed diploma scroll, a trophy or an artefact of some sort. It may be rationalised as being something they are proud of, something which symbolises achievement, or something they keep for show. The hardest thing of all to admit is that it is there because it has been imbued with any sort of magical or mystical significance.

Take the framed diploma, for example. True, it might be there on the wall to show clients that the diplomate is qualified and skilled. Its presence, however, is likely to have a subtle effect upon the diplomate. As long as it is there on the wall, it will seem to ensure success. Although it may be 'forgotten', or taken for granted, if it is removed the diplomate might experience some degree of upset, some sense of loss, some feeling of lessened skill. Essentially, the diploma had gradually been ascribed some magical significance.

In the context of Western Medicine we glibly talk about the phases of magic and religion, as if they are things of the past. This is just not the case. They may no longer be integral parts of medical practice, yet they are still there. We may no longer invoke the benevolence of a particular deity when an operation is performed or a prescription made out, yet there is not a surgeon or physician of any experience who has not silently asked for some sort of divine intervention in a difficult case. Whether they subscribe to a religion or not, somewhere deep within their minds they will believe and have asked for the aid of powers beyond their worldly experience.

In past times religion and magical beliefs were part and parcel of life. Nowadays we compartmentalise everything. As science and rationalism have become the dominant influences upon the way people are taught from childhood, so they learn to separate the different aspects of their lives. It is the 'place for everything and everything in its place' mentality. In a sense this can be a pretty efficient way of leading one's life. If you separate your religious beliefs from your work, then you by and large operate in the different spheres of your life according to different rules.

Let us take the example of a scientist who also happens to be deeply religious. In his job as an analyst he has to deal in facts and what he considers to be truths. In his spiritual life, on the other hand, he deals in belief because his religion demands acceptance of its doctrine. There is a potential conflict here. As a scientist he would realise that a belief is not necessarily based upon a truth. His training would tend to make him look for suitable tests to elucidate the truths of that religion. But, as long as he compartmentalises his science and his religion, he can avoid what could be a traumatic conflict.

Having said that, there is a conflict between magic, religion and science. Essentially, this is because magic and magical beliefs have in the past been outlawed by the dominant influence of religion. All practices which were considered to have no connection with the divine, were automatically labelled as being superstitions. And of course, living now in the dominant influence of science, whatever cannot be proven is considered false.

So basic is the belief in magic, however, that even although religion and science have rejected magical beliefs, they cannot and will not ever get rid of them. The 'gypsy remedies,' 'old wives tales' and 'rank superstitions' just keep bubbling away in that underground pool of Folk Medicine. From time to time they will burst to the surface and be tried out by ordinary people like you and me. It is inevitable, since deep down most people still do, and always will, believe in magic.

And of course it just may be that one day another great medical discovery will be fished out of that huge pool of underground knowledge.

The placebo – self-deception or magic?

Before science came along, people took medicines, remedies and recited charms whenever they felt ill. If they recovered they generally assumed that the medicine or charm had worked. Not an unreasonable assumption, one might think.

As medicine became more scientific, however, people began trying to find out precisely what was responsible in a treatment for making the individual better. Again, a perfectly laudable thing to do. Great advances were made. Out of the mish-mash of remedies with multiple ingredients it became possible to extract the single substance which was responsible for the improvement. Yet it did not prove to be quite so simple. It was discovered that sometimes patients improved when they were given a substance or treatment which was known to be ineffective.

As scientific drug trials became the common method of testing drugs, where an active drug was compared with a completely inert or inactive compound which looked exactly the same, this curious effect became more apparent. In innumerable studies it was found that about 40 per cent of people would respond positively to a *placebo,* as the inactive treatment was called (from the Latin *placere* – to please).

The *placebo effect* came to be regarded as a nuisance. Since up to 40 per cent of people can be expected to react to an inactive compound which they think is effective, it means that the researcher has to make allowances for this in a trial. Some researchers have even found that the percentage can be as high as 80 per cent!

The problem is that you cannot predict the so-called placebo response. You cannot say who is going to react positively to a placebo, because an individual may react on one occasion but not on the next, and vice versa. Countless studies have confirmed this.

We really know very little about the placebo. No-one has given a satisfactory explanation for it – and I doubt whether anyone ever will. It is, I believe, the scientific cop-out. When something cannot be explained, when a mechanism cannot be proven, then the placebo is invoked. All the Folk remedies of the past and many of the Complementary Medicines of the present are said to work simply by evoking a placebo response. Well, that may be the case, but it also has to be said that the placebo effect must be involved just as much in every type of treatment used in Medicine and Surgery. Again, there are ample studies which show that the more dramatic the treatment, the greater is the chance of a placebo reaction. Of course, there is no more dramatic procedure than a surgical operation.

I think it is true to say that science really misses the point of the placebo. Rather than writing it off as an unwanted phenomenon whereby people can be so gullible that they think an ineffective treatment is actually making them feel better (often dramatically), it should be the point of extensive research. What we see with the placebo is the process of self-healing. In some way the placebo, the treatment given, triggers off the body's natural healing mechanism. It is as simple as that.

Is the placebo effective because of an ingrained belief in magic? Or perhaps it is magic!

Magic and Folk Medicine

There are said to be three functions of magic, and three means of bringing the process of magic about. The functions are, production, destruction and protection. The means of bringing it about are through incantation, ritual and alteration of the practitioner's consciousness.

In the Folk Medicine context, only the functions of destruction and protection are of relevance. An illness or illness-producing factor is destroyed, or an illness, disease or accident is prevented by protecting the individual. Although one might say that the good health may be produced, this is not really part of the belief in Folk practice.

Not all three means of working magic are necessary at the same time. Indeed, as the practice of magic developed it divided into high and low magic. High magic depended more upon the alteration of consciousness of the practitioner. This could be achieved through drugs, chants, meditation, sleep deprivation, water deprivation and fasting. In a sense it became a religion of its own, driven underground by the forbidding attitude of orthodox religion. Low magic, on the other hand depended more upon ritual and incantation. It became the nature magic of rural communities, and the accepted manner of producing potions and medicines for centuries.

All three methods of bringing magic about can be found in Folk Medicine. In the shamanic tradition, from the North American Indian Medicine Man to his counterpart in far off Siberia, entering a state of trance is regarded as an integral part of the healing process. In these instances the Medicine Man is practising high magic.

Ritual and incantation are much commoner in the Folk Medicine practised by lay people. As we shall see, there is often quite interesting symbolism attached to the rituals.

Sympathetic or Transference Magic

In Folk Medicine one can see two distinct types of magic remedy. The treatment either depends upon sympathetic or transference magic.

Sympathetic Magic depends upon using something which is sympathetic, or very like the problem one is trying to solve. It may be that an animal, insect or plant was likened in some way to an illness, so would be considered of value if eaten, used in an ointment or applied in some such way. Many fertility remedies and aphrodisiacs were made according to this principle. Mandrake and bryony roots, being phallus-like were considered potency stimulators. So too were the genitalia of innumerable animals renowned for their 'potency'.

Another way in which sympathetic magic was used was when taking a compound or substance which produced symptoms which were like an illness. In such cases it was believed that if someone was afflicted with certain symptoms, they could be improved by using the magic of a herb or whatever to overcome the ill magic which was causing the illness. For example, a hallucinogenic fungus might be given to overcome hysteria or madness caused by evil spirits. Or a herb which caused sweating might be given to someone with a fever.

Transference magic depends upon using an object, plant or creature to take away the illness. For example, Culpepper tells us that to cure a wart one should take a black snail and rub it over the wart nine times in two directions. The snail should then be impaled upon a black-thorn. As it died, so would the wart waste away. Toothache and gum conditions were similarly cured by scratching the gum with a nail or piece of wood found in a graveyard. The nail was then hammered into a tree or the wood buried in an old grave. Either way, the pain was thought to be transferred from the sufferer.

Giving the illness to a creature, then allowing it to die was thus a common method of dealing with ailments. In the highlands of Scotland, if a live frog was placed in a bag and hung up a chimney, it was believed that as it croaked its last croak, it would cure a child of whooping cough.

Frogs were also used to cure thrush and other infections of the mouth. It was believed that if a live frog's head was placed in the sufferer's mouth, then dragged out by the legs and hurled as far away as possible, the infection would go with it. Snakes were also used to cure *wens*, or swellings in the throat (today, we would associate this with a thyroid goitre). A live snake was taken and drawn across the throat nine times, before being buried alive in a bottle. The theory was that as the snake died and decayed, so would the swelling reduce.

An ancient cure for epilepsy involved taking hair clippings and nail pairings and wrapping them up in a small bag together with a small coin, then burying them where three or four roads met, ie, at a crossroads. If they were picked up by some unfortunate passer-by, then it was hoped that the disease would transfer to them and mysteriously disappear from the sufferer.

Incantations – the importance of the spell

Every child knows that dock leaves are supposed to cure a nettle sting. Of course, when they try them out they find that they don't always work. The reason why, I was told many years ago, is because it only works when you say the words. The incantation, the actual spell is all important!

There are several variations of the nettle sting spell, a couple of samples being:–

" *Nettle in, dok out, now this, now that.*"

Geoffrey Chaucer (14th century)

"*In dockin leaf, nettle leave alain (alone)*"

Old Scottish charm

Burns, scalds and abrasions could apparently be dealt with by the following incantation:–

'*There came two angels from the north.*
One was fire and one was frost.
Out, fire! In frost!
In the name of the Father, Son and Holy Ghost.'

In the Middle Ages St Blaise, the patron saint of wool-combers, was often invoked when one had been wounded by a thorn, the tooth of a comb or a splinter. One simply covered the wound with a hand and said:–

'*Blaise, the martyr, commands thee to come forth,*
In the Name of the Lord Jesus Christ.'

In general the incantation, or charm was used in combination with a ritual. In the nettle cure, the ritual was the way in which the dock leaf was screwed up to bruise the leaf, then rubbed over the area of sting. More serious injuries often had more structured rituals and more complicated incantations.

For example, to treat an Adder (snake) bite, two pieces of hazel wood had to be placed across the bite in the shape of a cross while the following incantation was sung:–

"*Underneath this hazelin mote,*
There's a maggoty worm with a speckled throat.
Nine double is he;.
And from nine double to eight double,
And from eight double to seven double.........

and continuing until:–

> *And from One double to no double,*
> *No double hath he."*

And this was supposed to reduce the swelling and reduce any effect of the poison.

You will note that the incantation involved the number nine. This was because numbers played a very important part in magic. In particular, the numbers three and nine recur in Folk Medicine rituals whereby the individual has to repeat a routine three or nine times. For example, to cure certain chronic conditions the sufferer often had to be passed through an aperture of some sort, whether a holed stone, under the belly of a standing animal or between designated boulders, either three or nine times depending upon the local custom. This was considered to be a sort of re-birthing, which was sanctified by doing it the appropriate number of times.

Three was considered mystical in the East and the West. It was, after all considered a sign of the Trinity. Nine, being a multiple of three, was considered a particularly powerful number.

In Devon, sciatica used to be called *boneshave*. To cure it, a sufferer had to go to a river and act out the following little ritual and incantation. While lying beside the river, preferably one flow-ing Southwards, with a stout stick between him and the river, he had to cry out:–

> *"Boneshave right, boneshave straight,*
> *As the water runs by the stave, good for boneshave."*

The Evil Eye – a need for protection

The fear that some people are capable of exerting a malign influence on others just by looking at them, by their having the Evil Eye, has been universal since the beginning of recorded history. People have believed that gypsies, witches, sorcerers and medicine men have acquired this ability, while some people are born with it. The problem is that people are not always aware

MAGIC AND MEDICINE · *29*

of who has put the Evil Eye on them, until they start to become ill.

The Evil Eye was described in cuneiform texts from Ancient Babylon as long ago as 3,000 BC. It was also known to the Ancient Egyptians, the Greeks and the Romans. Today, it is known as *mal occhia* in Italy, *mal de ojo* in Spain, *ayn* in Arabic cultures, and *casm-e-sur* in Iran. It still holds fear for people right across the globe.

Whenever an individual feels that they have been given the Evil Eye, there is a need to counteract it. Advocated methods are to spit, make the sign of the *fig* (the closed fist with the thumb inside), or for a man, to clutch his genitals. Alternatively, the Evil Eye can be averted by using an amulet or talisman.

Talismanic magic

Amulets and talismans have been used since prehistoric times. The roots of many which are made, distributed and bought today can be traced back to Antiquity.

Although people often imagine that the two terms mean the same thing, they are actually quite different.

A *Talisman* is an object of some sort which has been specially constructed for a particular purpose. As such there is a definite magical aim involving a ritual and incantation as the object is prepared, usually under particular astrological influences. It is an active magical device.

An *Amulet*, on the other hand, is usually a smaller, portable object which is believed to protect or ward off evil, bewitchment or the malign influence of the Evil Eye. The name is derived from an Arab root, meaning to carry.

Another term often confused with these is a *Charm*. Essentially, these are simple devices whose purpose is merely to give the carrier good luck. These are things like the traditional rabbit's foot, the lump of coal, the four-leaf clover.

In Folk Medicine the difference between these terms has become blurred over the years. Many of the oldest talismans can be bought as good luck charms or as charms for keeping the owner healthy. In addition, there are still many everyday objects which are imbued with a magical significance when found in particular situations. For example, a pin found upon the ground is associated with the old saying:

> "*See a pin, pick it up;*
> *All the day you'll have good luck.*"

In the same way, a four-leaf clover found by chance while out on a walk would bring fortune in different aspects of one's life. Thus:

> "*One leaf for fame,*
> *And one for wealth*
> *A third for a faithful lover,*
> *Yet another to bring you glorious health,*
> *And all in a four-leaf clover.*"

The scarab, or beetle, is an extremely common Ancient Egyptian amulet which was used as a general health charm and as a specific aid to enhance fertility. It was the symbol of the god Khepri, the Lord of Transformations who was thought to roll the sun across the heavens in order to turn night into day. The humble dung-beetle which rolled its eggs in a ball of dung was taken to be a microcosmic representation of the god's activity. Since Khepri was also considered a healing deity, the act of rolling a ball was imitated in the preparation of medications. Thus, it is likely that the pill was invented from this religico-magical background in the second millenia BC. And this is a matter of considerable significance, since the pill is the medical equivalent to the discovery of the wheel.

The scarab's fertility link has subsequently passed across the world. Beetles have been worn as amulets by childless women in different countries over many centuries. Indeed, as a piece of sympathetic magic they have been included in remedies to enhance fertility in Greece, the Mediterranean countries and Britain.

The Eye of Horus (Figure 3) is another Egyptian amulet commonly used to guard against the Evil Eye and bewitchment. It is commonly seen on pendants and rings across the whole of Europe.

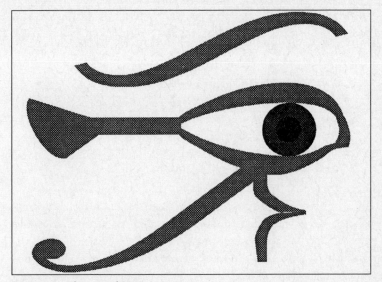

Figure 3   The eye of Horus

The Ptolemaic Period of Egyptian history, as mentioned in the last chapter, resulted in the amalgamation of Egyptian, Persian and Greek beliefs. The spread of their empires and the subsequent rise of Rome, carried the germs of talismanic magic to the far corners of the Ancient world.

The spread of the cult of the Egyptian goddess Isis, carried *the symbol of the moon crescent* far and wide. Ancient Greek and Roman women wore moon-shaped buckles on their shoes to prevent the 'moon-madness' and the cyclical changes of nature brought about by the influence of the moon. Here, we may be seeing one of the earliest references to the premenstrual syndrome.

Some authorities suggest that *the horseshoe* is directly linked to the crescent moon symbol of Isis. It is recorded that it was nailed to the doors of houses by the Romans as a protection against the Plague and the Evil Eye. It was, of course, used in the same manner centuries later in Britain, although by then it may have been associated with the christianised tale that St Dunstan nailed the shoe to the devil's single hoof and caused such pain that he dared not look upon a horseshoe again. Interestingly, the Christian link was also mixed with a Scandinavian theme in another incantation which had to be sung while nailing the horseshoe to a door:

> *"Father, Son and Holy Ghost*
> *Nail the devil to this post,*
> *Thrice I smites with Holy Crook,*
> *With this mell I thrice do knock,*
> *One for God,*
> *And one for Wod,*
> *And one for Lok."*

While it might be supposed that 'Wod' and 'Lok' could be mis-spellings of wood and lock, it is suggested by some authorities that the words respectively stand for Woden or Odin, the Norse King of the Gods, and Loki, another teutonic deity.

The Celts were skilled amulet makers before the Romans arrived in Britain. A veritable industry thrived for centuries in Ireland and the highlands of Scotland. With the wealth of semi-precious stones and a skill in metal-working, Celtic amulets, sure-cures against the Evil Eye, were exported abroad in great numbers.

Unfortunately, the Ancient Celts did not leave us a written legacy. Most of our knowledge of them has come from written accounts by the Romans and other societies who had dealings with them. Their art and their rich mythology, however, still continue to influence people today.

The coming of Christianity introduced the belief that certain saints could cure particular conditions. Accordingly, relics of the saints or amulets dedicated to them became part of Folk Medicine.

Saints Cosmas and Damian, the 'holy brothers,' were 3rd century physicians who became the patron saints of the healing professions. St Dunstan and St Thomas became the protectors of eyes and were invoked for healing of eye problems. St Teresa of Avila, reputed to have been shot through the heart by an angel's arrow, became the patron saint of heart victims. St Dympna of Gheel became the patron saint of the insane and was invoked against mental illness and epilepsy. St Agatha of Catania in Sicily was the patron saint of wet nurses and considered to be a power-ful aid in diseases of the breast and for childless couples. St Timothy of Lystra, a disciple of Paul, became the patron of stomach disease. Similarly, St Rocco, who treated Plague victims, and St Elizabeth who treated lepers, became associated with these specific illnesses. Their very names etched or written on amulets were believed to offer some protection.

St Blaise, the earlier-mentioned patron of wool-combers was also the patron saint of sore throats. Ever since the 16th century, sore throat sufferers have been invited to take the blessing of St Blaise. This involves placing two candles upon the throat, since the saint is always portrayed as holding two candles.

St Antony the Hermit (of Thebes) was believed to be able to intervene in cases of the devastating illness *St Antony's Fire*. This was a condition which caused toxicity, raging temperature and progressive gangrene. It has subsequently been found to be due to the fungus ergot which grows on rye, which was of course used to make bread. His amulet took the form of a **T-shaped cross**, which incidentally is common in many religions. He was also apparently skilled in treating Erysipelas (now known to be caused by a bacterial infection) and epilepsy, for which his amulets were also used to protect against.

An extremely popular charm against evil, accident and disease was the Cross of St Benedict (Figure 4). This consisted of a blessing inscribed in abbreviated form upon and around the cross. It would generally have been worn as a medallion. Each letter stood for a word. They were arranged so that the four letters in the angles of the cross stood for the first four words of the first line. The letters of the upright of the cross, from top to bottom, stood for the second line, followed by the horizontal for the third line. And finally, the rest of the blessing was arranged around the outside.

The blessing was in Latin:–

Crux Sancti Patris Benedicte.
Crux Sancta sit mihi lux.
Ne daemon sit mihi dux.
Vade retro Satana,
Ne suade mihi vana:
Sunt mala quae libas,
Ipse venena bibas.

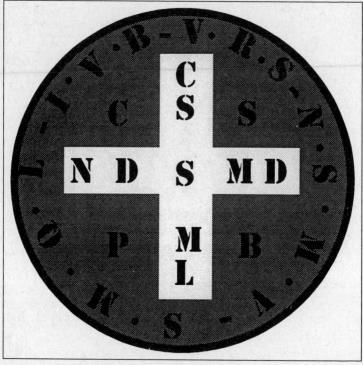

Figure 4   St Benedict's Cross

In translation this means:–

> *Cross of the Holy Father Benedict.*
> *Holy Cross be my light.*
> *Let no evil spirit be my guide.*
> *Get thee behind me Satan,*
> *Suggest no vain delusions:*
> *What thou offerest is evil,*
> *Thou thyself drinkest poison.*

Related to relics of saints was the belief in the magic of the earth itself. In particular, the earth walked on by saints, the earth from burial sites and the earth from places where three or four lands or roads met (crossroads).

The Romans highly valued sealed earth from Arezzo, which they called *Terra sigillata*. They believed it to be useful against all plagues and poisoning. In Britain in later centuries a similar use was made for it against consumption.

Carrying graveyard soil or tombstone moss in a small bag hung round the neck was effective in warding off the Evil Eye and in protecting the carrier against rheumatism and agues.

The material of coffins was also frequently used to make health charms. They were supposed to have been dug up in order to work best. Coffin handles, nails and hinges were all thought to alleviate cramp pains anywhere in the body when made into a ring. In addition, an old highland belief was that the metal from a decomposed coffin worn as a medallion would cure epilepsy, and prevent gout and rheumatism.

It was not only saints who were believed to have the ability to cure. Kings and Emperors were supposedly able to cure people. According to Tacitus, the Emperor Vespasian performed many miraculous cures at Alexandria. In England, King Edward the Confessor began a long tradition of the *Royal Touch*, when he was recorded as healing cases of *scrofula*, otherwise known as the *King's Evil*, back in the year 1058. This was a mixed bag of conditions whereby the sufferer presented with glandular suppurating swellings. It should be clear that under this blanket term there would have been a whole host of conditions from the simple, trivial and curable, to the chronic, malignant and incurable.

At first the Kings and Queens of England actually did have occasions when they would physically touch people to facilitate the cure. Inevitably, though, this arduous task was eased by the making of talismans to do the job. By doing this it was possible to distribute the talismans to various parts of the country where sufferers could make a pilgrimage to. Significantly, the original talisman used was a ring which had been brought back from Jerusalem by Edward the Confessor.

These talismans, called *touch pieces*, were specially minted as coins or rings. Then they were placed in a dish and had a prayer of healing said over them. After that, the King or Queen would take them in their hands and rub them, while saying:–

"Sanctify, O Lord, these rings and graciously bedew them with the dew of thine benediction and consecration, and hallow them by the rubbing of our hands which thou hast been pleased according to our ministry, to the end that what the nature of the metal is not able to perform may be wrought by the greatness of thy grace."

The most famous of all the Middle Ages talismans was the word *ABRACADABRA*. It was apparently first referred to by the Roman physician, Severus Sammonicus in the second century AD. Its power in the popular imagination was such that it survived for centuries, and is still used today in lay parlance as the best known of all the magic words of power.

To have the best effect the letters were to be written on parchment, as in Figure 5, then worn around the neck for nine days. At that time it was to be hurled backwards while it was still dark, preferably into a stream which was running Eastwards.

It was thought to be particularly effective against the Plague, but

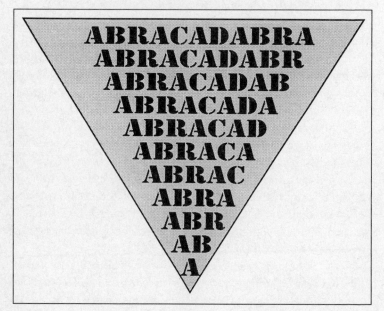

Figure 5

all other ailments could be dealt with by it. Indeed, for the simple relief of rheumatism, it was suggested that the word be repeated again and again, dropping a letter from the beginning on each occasion.

Various stones have been used in Folk Medicine over the years. Huge holed stones, such as the *Men-an-Tol* in Cornwall, were used to treat sufferers from rickets, scrofula and epilepsy. The naked person was passed through the hole nine times in order to *re-birth* the individual. Other similar stones around the country were used in the same ritual manner.

Small holed pebbles, called *witch-stones* when I was a boy, were used as necklaces, bangles or medallions to keep evil spirits and witches spells away. These have been common around the entire world for centuries.

Elf-shot, the name given to flint arrow-heads, commonly believed to be fired by elves, were used as amulets in past days. They were regarded as protection against the Evil Eye, provided they were never allowed to drop to the ground once they had been discovered. Thus, people wore them around their necks. Sometimes, they were dipped in water, an ill person drinking from the cup being promised relief from their illness.

Crystals, gems and semi-precious stones have all been used as amulets. The following *birth-stones* have been used in Folk Medicine for many years. While not being specifically Zodiacal stones, they are manufactured and bought according to the month of the individuals's birth. They are also thought to have beneficial effects with certain conditions.

JANUARY – GARNET – active against infections and depression.

FEBRUARY – AMETHYST – blood disorders, sleep difficulties, anxiety and ill-effects of alcohol.

MARCH – BLOODSTONE – for liver and kidney disorders.

APRIL – DIAMOND – infections, evil influences, mental fatigue.

MAY – EMERALD – eye problems , sleep problems.

JUNE – AGATE – self-confidence, gum problems, bites and poisoning.

JULY – RUBY – arthritis, cramps and spasms.

AUGUST – SARDONYX – gives self-control and balance in all things.

SEPTEMBER – SAPPHIRE – bleeding problems, anxiety.

OCTOBER – OPAL – lung problems and digestive disorders.

NOVEMBER – TOPAZ – throat problems, protects against evil influences.

DECEMBER – TURQUOISE – a tonic stone, particularly good at helping the nervous and those who hate speaking in public. The old saying goes:

> *"If you wear a turquoise blue,*
> *Success will crown whate'er you do."*

In general, the above stones are said to work best for those born in those months, although they are said to help the disorders mentioned. However, it is said they must not be bought by the individual, but must be bought as a gift for them!

Some other substances, thought to be 'stones' have been used extensively in rural areas over the years. In the highland moors of Scotland, where adders were common, so-called *Adder stones* were eagerly sought after. These were thought to have been produced by the concretion of adder spit. Small Adder stones were believed to be effective against snake-bites, eye problems and the whooping cough in children.

Eagle Stones, thought to have been stones left by eagles in their nests to ensure fertility, were imported in quantity from the East in the 17th and 18th centuries. They were thought to aid both pregnancy and labour when worn about the neck.

Bezoar Stones, concretions found in the stomachs of ruminant animals all over the world – such as cattle, antelopes, goats and llamas – have been used as both amulets against the Evil Eye, and as ingredients in love potions, poison antidotes and in various internal medicines.

Toadstones, were similar to Adder stones, in that they were hard concretions thought to have come from the heads of very old toads. They were thought to be effective against witches, sorcerers, the Evil Eye, as well as being important ingredients in love potions. It was said that the authenticity of a toadstone could be checked by confronting a live toad with the stone. If it was genuine, the toad would come towards it, as if to gain it.

Many other charms and amulets were made from animal materials. Most of them are good examples of sympathetic and transference magic.

The foot of a mole, if cut off while the poor animal was still living, was used in many parts of England as a cure for toothache when worn as an amulet.

Pliny, writing in AD 77 tells us that the tooth from a mole was also useful for toothache when it was worn attached to the clothing. He also wrote that a rabbit or hare's foot could cure gout and cramp.

In many parts of England and Scotland people used to (and still do) carry *cramp bones*. These could be the patella or knuckle-bone of a sheep, or hare. Worn as an amulet they were supposed to protect one from the cramp pains of rheumatism and gout. Placed under the pillow they were believed to cure all sorts of muscular pains overnight.

In Yorkshire, England, the wearing of an *eel-skin garter* was (and still is) advocated in rural areas to prevent and cure cramp and rheumatism. It was hoped that the suppleness of the eel would transfer itself to the afflicted joint.

Snake-skins were also used throughout the country as cures for all sorts of puncturing wounds. They were considered a specific remedy for thorn wounds. Not only that, but as headbands or hat bands they were thought to prevent or cure headaches.

The skins of long-chested animals, such as *hares*, were thought to be capable of transfering the lung-efficiency of the animal to an asthma sufferer. The skin was simply placed over the sufferer's chest while they slept.

Mice and shrews were thought to carry all sorts of ailments, particularly lameness. Carrying a live shrew in a box or pot about the neck, until it died was a remedy of Antiquity which was used to cure lameness, paralysis and apoplexy (strokes).

Similarly, *spiders* were thought to be useful in getting rid of coughs. An old remedy was to place a live spider in a matchbox and wear it around the neck. As the spider died, so was the cough supposed to disappear.

A particularly powerful amulet which has been used throughout the world, from the days of the Classical Greeks until almost the present day, is *the caul*. This is the name given to the membranes which surround the foetus in the womb. Sometimes a child is born with the membranes partially or completely intact. In parts of Italy it was believed that the child born wearing *il velo della Madonna*, the veil of Madonna, would as an adult have the power to nullify evil and cure diseases by making the sign of the cross against them.

As a protection against drowning, however, the caul achieved universal fame. Sailors and fishermen would be prepared to spend considerable amounts to buy one to protect them while at sea. And incidentally, it was believed that the man who carried one would never suffer from sea-sickness or scurvy.

Mystical Plants

Herbs and other plants have formed the bedrock for most medical systems throughout the world since the beginning of civilisation. Modern medicine is continually extracting and developing new drugs from plant sources, often confirming the medical uses which the Ancients ascribed to them. Some plants, however, have been used simply because they were believed to possess some mystical power of their own.

The Assyro-Babylonians and the Egyptians venerated the *pomegranate*. Garlands were woven from its blooms, its fragrance was used in perfumed oils, a drink was made from its red juice, and a healing salve was prepared from the root. The Egyptians considered it an essential plant to be taken into the afterlife.

The Romans used to fill their homes with *laurel and bay* leaves during the month of January. This of course was the month named after their god Janus, the deity with two heads who presided over doorways, entrances, and beginnings and ends. His two faces looked in opposite directions, one to the past and the other to the future. At the beginning of the year Janus, Apollo and Aesculapius were invoked to keep the household free of sickness and disease, hence the laurel and bay leaves which were sacred to Apollo and his son Aesculapius, the god of Medicine.

The Druids worshipped the *oak* and were said to perform their ceremonies in oak groves. It is believed that the oak was especially significant to them because the mistletoe grew upon it. During the winter solstice mistletoe was ceremonially cut from the oak boughs by Druid priests and then used in the making of healing remedies. It was believed that it could remove the wrath of the gods, thereby being used as a cure for epilepsy, St.Vitus's Dance and madness.

The *Rowan Tree*, or Mountain Ash, has always had a significance to the Scots. It was believed to protect from the Evil Eye and guard against witches and bewitchment. Perhaps it is for this reason that people of Scottish ancestry unconsciously plant such a tree in their gardens (as indeed did the author!)

Ivy was another plant grown on Roman houses. It was dedicated to the god Bacchus and was thought to protect the dwellers from poverty and depressed spirits.

Mandrake is perhaps the most famous of all magico-medical plants. It was used by the Assyro-Babylonians and the Egyptians as a narcotic agent and was used in Biblical times as told in Genesis 30, 14.

The Romans used it as a hypnotic, a painkiller and an eye treatment. A manuscript from that time describes how it should be pulled from the ground by a black dog while the man protected his ears from the mandrake's shrieking as it was pulled from the ground. It was believed that the shriek would turn a man mad and that disease and death would come to the creature that drew its roots from the soil.

In later times the mandrake root was used in aphrodisiacs, cough cures and as general amulets against the Evil Eye. It was also believed that for a mandrake to be truly effective it had to be one which had grown underneath a gallows where a man had been hanged. It was said that the matter which fell to the ground from the body caused the plant to take on the form of a man. And the more man-like the plant root was, the more powerful was the root's magic.

Healing Vessels

Throughout history it has been believed that the vessels in which medicines were given could actually store up a sort of magic, which would render the medicine more effective.

In primitive cultures it was thought that a vanquished enemy's skull could prove to be not only a powerful talisman, but also a potential healing vessel. To drink from a cup fashioned from the cranium was thought to give the drinker the strength of the vanquished foe.

The *human skull* was also thought to be a potent healing vessel for those afflicted by epilepsy. According to the Roman historian Pliny, epilepsy could be cured by drinking spring water at night from the skull of a slain man.

This use of the skull recurs again and again across Europe. Indeed, not only was it believed that drinking from a skull was curative, but that if food was cooked in it, virtually any disease could be relieved.

Animal horn, particularly the mythical *unicorn horn*, was thought to make a particularly good healing vessel. In fact, most of the so-called unicorn horns of the past were derived from the tusk of the narwhal, one of the toothed dolphins.

Tortoise shell was commonly used to make goblets, medicine cups and spoons.

Its particular range of activity was over female problems and fertility treatments. In addition, because of the great age to which tortoises lived, it was considered an ideal healing vessel material from which to drink tonics 'to keep one going.'

Shells were used throughout the world. In particular, *Mother-of-Pearl* was thought to be especially good for strengthening the heart and for dealing with feverish conditions.

Gold was of course a material much favoured by the wealthy for its healing properties. A golden goblet was considered to be effective against leprosy and jaundice, and protective to the heart and blood.

Silver being associated with the moon was thought to be useful against female tantrums, depression, madness, as well as being useful in dealing with the pains of menstruation.

Quartz crystal, because of its sparkle, was thought to be effective against eye disorders, scrofula, heart and stomach problems.

Chapter Three

Medical Divination

'The hand is the organ of organs, the active agent
of the passive powers of the entire system.

Aristotle

'There is some ill a-brewing towards my rest,
For I did dream of money-bags tonight.'

William Shakespeare
The Merchant of Venice

Divination, the process of foretelling, has always been part
of Folk Medicine. It was, of course, also part of established
Medicine until the scientific method was introduced. Yet
even now, in a sense, divination is part of the process of diagnosis.
It is true that technology has given us the ability to see into the body
with X-rays, Magnetic Resonance Intensifiers and Computerised
Axial Tomography, yet even these highly sophisticated methods do
not always give us a full answer. They take the doctor a long way
down the path towards finding the answer, but sometimes that just
means that his best-guess, his divination of the problem is made
from a broader knowledge base. There is still plenty of room for
error.

Now I am not making any criticism of modern Medicine here.
As a doctor I am grateful for the advances which technological
Medicine has brought to patient care. What I am saying is that

despite all of the sophisticated equipment and techniques now at our disposal, diagnosis is nowhere near a precise science. At the end of the day, after all the tests and investigations, an individual still has to make a decision. When the answer evades him or her, then intuition may be brought to bear. In other words, even in the most refined temples of knowledge, our teaching hospitals, the art of medical divination still goes on.

Back in the days of the Assyro-Babylonians diseases were thought to be the result of some supernatural cause brought upon the individual as a punishment for sin. Diagnosis was pure divination then. Animals were sacrificed and their entrails examined. This method, called *hepatoscopy*, primarily focused upon the appearance of the liver of the sacrificial animal. As evidence of this method, several clay models of livers complete with divinatory markings have been found by archaeologists.

The Romans had absorbed much of the scientific knowledge of the Greeks, but still believed widely in a supernatural element in illness. Indeed, it is known that as far back as the seventh century BC there was a college of Augurs in Rome. The Augurs were priests specially trained in the divinatory arts. Virtually every disease was associated with a particular deity. Through reading omens, casting horoscopes, and various mantic methods they divined the problem and advised upon the most appropriate way of propitiating the gods.

Basically, health omens fell into three main groups:- disease, recovery or death. Many of those omens have survived in Folk Medicine to this day.

Omens of disease

Omens are really just events or happenings which are thought to be indicative of things to come.

Bats flying over one's home during the day were considered a sign of forthcoming disease.

Crows, ravens and jackdaws which hover directly over a person and squawk noisily are considered a sign of impending illness.

Hares are considered to be ill omens, particularly to do with mobility or breathing. If an individual suddenly disturbs one, then it can indicate a chest problem or some problem which might befall the individual's limbs, possibly an accident.

Owls hooting in the grounds of one's home were thought to herald the onset of illness within the home.

Rats or mice getting into one's home and nibbling at clothes was a sure sign of illness on its way.

Worms or slugs entering one's house implied that some infectious ailment might be imminent.

Omens of recovery

Often these would be a reverse of the omens of disease. Thus, crows or jackdaws leaving their nests would indicate that they were taking the illness away, or that the illness would follow. Similarly, when birds, insects or things started to rise, it might be indicative of a lifting of the condition. Thus, swarms of insects flying up, a flock of birds rising from the vicinity or smoke rising straight upwards were all taken as signs that recovery was starting to take place.

Signs of increased energy were also thought to indicate healing. The sudden foaming of an opened beer bottle, the spurting out of a hot coal from the fire, a spraying from a tap have all been recorded as good recovery omens.

Omens of death

In days gone-by most people knew of these omens and feared them. In a sense this was understandable, since death rates were higher and terminal illnesses came and carried off relatively young people with frightening speed.

Death-watch beetles were always considered ominous signs. They are destructive of furniture and woodwork and used to be found in musty environments. The clicking noise was produced by the insect knocking its head against the wood.

Magpies are also associated with death, but only if a single one is seen.

Falling ornaments, particularly those to do with an individual used to be well known signs of death or doom. A picture or portrait which fell to the floor of its own accord had to be replaced immediately and the sign countered by the use of an amulet or the sign of the cross.

A *howling dog* is another omen which seems pretty well universal as a sign of death. There are countless examples throughout history, one of the most famous being to do with the so-called Curse of Tutankhamen.

Throughout the Winter of 1922 the world waited with bated breath as Howard Carter and Lord Carnarvon gradually cleared the entrance to the tomb of Tutankhamen in the Valley of the Kings. At the tomb entrance were the words:–

'The wings of death will surely strike him who disturbs the peace of the dead Pharaoh.'

The 'Curse' was of course ignored and on 17th February 1923 the burial chamber was officially opened. On the 6th March Lord Carnarvon was bitten by a mosquito upon his left cheek. The bite became infected and he developed pneumonia and septicaemia. At 1.55am on the 5th April, in a Cairo hotel, he died. At exactly the same time, all of the lights in Cairo went out. Most amazingly, however, at the same time back in his England home, Lord Carnarvon's pet labrador started howling.

Then it too died.

When the Pharoah's mummy was subsequently unwrapped, a tiny scar was also found upon the left cheek, corresponding to that of Carnarvon.

Dreams

The interpretation of dreams was one of the earliest preoccupations of healers. The Ancient Greeks had sleep temples dedicated to a variety of gods who presided over this most mystical aspect of a person's life. There was *Hypnos*, the god of sleep; *Thanatos*, his twin brother and the god of death; *Oneiros*, the god of dreams and *Hermes*, the messenger of the gods who brought messages from Zeus to men as they slept.

Oneiromancy, the art of dream interpretation was an integral part of early medical practices. Its popularity and the degree to which it has been accepted by orthodoxy has been variable over the succeeding centuries. The late nineteenth and the twentieth centuries have seen a re-awakening of the subject as successive psychiatrists such as Freud, Jung and Adler have opened up the field.

It is outside the scope of a book on Folk Medicine to explore the nature of sleep and dreams. Indeed, the actual theories have little to do with the way that the symbolism of dreams have drifted into the pool of folk knowledge. The fact is that they have, and that there are many Folk Medicine 'practitioners' who are probably just as adept in dream interpretation as their professional orthodoxly trained counterparts.

Let us take a swift look at some dream symbology which has been drawn from the pool of Folk Medicine.

Abandoned – to dream of being abandoned and lost is thought to indicate that one is in a precarious state of health and that great care needs to be taken, particularly when exposed to physical danger or infections.

Abyss – a common 'falling' dream. Again, it indicates a time of vulnerability.

Accident – if one dreams of an accident while travelling or contemplating travel then this is thought to be a warning not to go, since life or limb might be at serious risk.

Ageing – to see oneself at an older age indicates a pending illness. To see others ageing indicates that one is getting better. The same applies to seeing oneself at a younger age.

Alligator – to dream of this or a crocodile indicates physical danger.

Baby – to dream of a baby indicates recovery from illness.

Bath – indicates guilt and the need to wash away one's sins.

Bats – indicate ill fortune, possibly in health.

Bells – tolling bells imply that someone close may die.

Birds – injured birds or birds with clipped or broken wings imply depression or mental strife.

Blindness – this indicates physical problems for others. If the dreamer is blind then there may be emotional or sexual problems.

Blood – to dream of blood indicates an imbalance in one's health which needs to be rectified by losing body fluids.

Buried alive – a dream of anxiety. Can indicate chest problems and breathing problems.

Candle – indicates a pregnancy for someone close. The holder of the candle may be involved.

Clock – to see a clock or hear it strike is a sign of someone's death.

Coffin – indicates a death to someone close.

Crossroads – indicates a major decision or a crisis in health.

Dead – to dream of the dead is a good health sign. It implies sure recovery from illness and good health thereafter.

Dogs – if howling indicate a death to someone close.

Drowning – implies that the individual is struggling and wants to be 'reborn' to have another go.

Fire – a sexual dream. It indicates that there might be a problem with sexual matters.

Food – dreaming of unpleasant food indicates a nauseous problem, perhaps to do with stomach disorders.

Goat – to dream of a black goat indicates physical illness. A dream of a white goat is a sexual dream.

Horses – generally a sexual dream.

Killing – to dream that one is killing someone or some creature is a sign of improvement in one's condition. It is like a safety valve for suppressed anger.

King – this usually represents one's father. The state of health of the king indicates if there is a problem.

Knives – represent danger.

Locks – indicate confusion. The individual needs help, someone to help them find the key to their problem.

Licking – this indicates a need to feel close to someone. It might be a sign of depression. Alternatively, it can be a sexual dream if enjoyed.

Nurses – to dream of nurses or doctors implies good health or a return to health.

Owl – to dream of a hooting owl may indicate coming illness or death to a close person.

Paralysis – to dream of being paralysed and unable to move is indicative of fear about a mobility problem or developing rheumatism or arthritis.

Queen – indicates the individual's mother. The state of health of the mother indicates the problem.

Rainstorm – with thunder and lightning implies mental distress, or approaching anxieties.

Rats – indicate an infectious illness.

Smoke – indicates confusion and a need for help.

Snake – this indicates healing, as it is the traditional sign of healing.

Toad – if the dream is associated with nausea, it indicates a stomach problem or a skin problem.

Tunnel – thought to represent a birth trauma. Similar to the dream of being buried alive.

Water – generally, all water dreams are to do with sexual desires. In older people they may be associated with urinary problems.

Not all dream analysts will agree with the above listing, but it has to be pointed out that there is no specific interpretation with any dream. The above listing is based upon commonly held beliefs.

Astrology

Astrology has been practised since the dawn of civilisation. Different systems were devised by the Babylonians, Egyptians, Chinese, Mayans and the Ancient Indians. Elements of all of these methods are still practised throughout the world today. At the heart of all Astrology is the belief that the movements of the planets against the backdrop of the stars, particularly the Zodiac belt, affect events, happenings and people on Earth. Even more than that, there is a belief that man, the microcosm, mirrors the universe, the macrocosm.

Astrology, as one of the first sciences known to man, was inevitably an integral part of magico-medicine. Since each individual occupied a unique position in the universe at any one time, the influences of the universe pattern upon him would also be unique to him. For centuries Astrology was taught as part of the curriculum in medical schools, it being considered essential that a physician should consider the patient as part of the universe, and his illness and treatment influenced by the apparent movement of heavenly bodies.

Nowadays, thanks to popular Astrology in newspapers and

magazines, virtually everyone knows their 'Sun sign.' This is the Zodiacal sign against which the Sun could be seen at the moment of the individual's birth. An important aspect of the Sun sign is that each one has an influence over a different part of the body. This is a very old concept dating from the days of the second century Roman Astrologer and mathematician Claudius Ptolemy. His original descriptions of Zodiacal associations came to be depicted as *Melothesic, or Astrological Man* (Figure 6).

Essentially, the Sun signs were associated with the body as follows:–

ARIES – the brain and head.
TAURUS – the throat.
GEMINI – the shoulders and arms and upper nervous system.
CANCER – the rib cage and breasts.
LEO – the heart and upper back.
VIRGO – the stomach and upper abdominal organs.
LIBRA – the kidneys, back and pelvis.
SCORPIO – the reproductive organs and bladder.
SAGITTARIUS – the hips, thighs and sciatic nerve.
CAPRICORN – the knees and the skin.
AQUARIUS – ankles and the lower leg, lower leg veins.
PISCES – the feet and the eyes.

Many people are also aware of the fact that when they cast a horoscope Astrologers divide the sky into twelve segments, which are called Houses. Each House is said to be concerned with a different aspect of the individual's life. The first House (which in popular Astrology corresponds with the Sun sign) is associated with the ego and personality of the person. The fourth House has to do with the home, and the sixth House is to do with the individual's health. A glance at Figure 7 will enable the reader to calculate their sixth House, which will show additional parts of the body which might prove troublesome. The Sun sign should be considered the first House, so that the health House will be the sixth. For example, with a Libra Sun sign the sixth House will be Pisces. Hence their potential trouble areas are the kidneys, lower back, eyes and the feet.

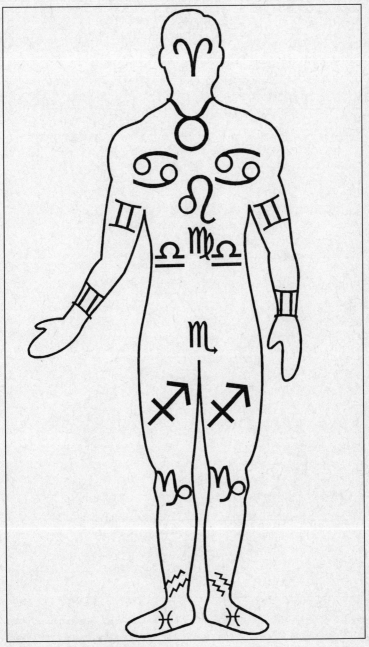

Figure 6   Astrological Man

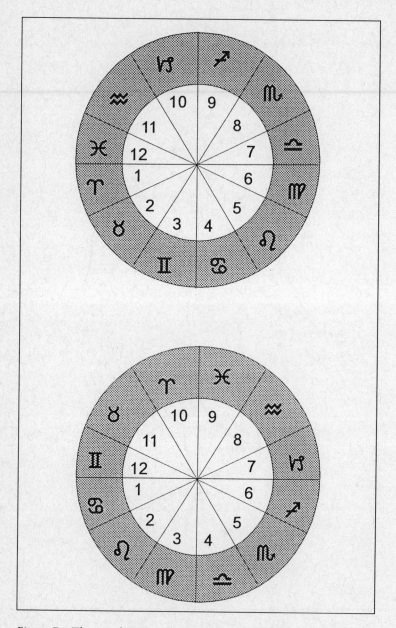

Figure 7 *The top diagram shows that for an Aries sun sign the sixth House would be Virgo. The bottom diagram shows that for a Cancer sun sign the sixth House would be Sagittarius.*

In addition, the planets are also said to affect different parts and functions of the body. The combination of all these principles in a horoscope, according to Medical Astrologers, brings an added dimension to treatment.

Each sign is said to be associated with its own herbal or plant remedies. Examples are:–

Aries – mint.
Taurus – centaury.
Gemini – valerian.
Cancer – ribwort.
Leo – common nettle.
Virgo – liquorice.
Libra – meadowsweet.
Scorpio – yarrow.
Sagittarius – sage.
Capricorn – comfrey.
Aquarius – ginger.
Pisces – elecampane.

Palmistry

Like Astrology, Palmistry has been practised by people in different cultures for several millennia. Also, like Astrology it was considered an integral part of medical practice and was taught in medical schools and universities for centuries. Plato, Anaxagoras and Galen all wrote about the markings of the hand when studying man, while Hippocrates, Aristotle and Paracelsus all extolled the virtue of reading the palm in making a diagnosis. It is still a recognised part of some established medical systems throughout the world. Indeed, recent research published in the British Medical Journal has indicated that certain skin creases and whorl patterns are predictors of circulatory problems including high blood pressure. Further research may well confirm some of the older teachings.

Palmistry is common in Folk Medicine practice. Many people dabble in the art and have a passing fair knowledge of the subject. There are, in fact, several branches of Palmistry. *Chirognomy* is the study of character through hand analysis; *Chirosophy* is the comparative study of hands; and *Chiromancy* is the study of fortune-telling by hand reading. Palmistry as practised in Folk Medicine draws on all three branches, albeit in an unsystemised manner.

The colour of the hand is thought to tell about the character of the individual. Thus, pink palms and hands indicate warm, sympathetic and healthy people. Red palms and hands indicate toughness both physically and mentally. Pale hands show coldness, aloofness and a tendency to depression.

The shape of the hand is said to tell about character. Thus, rectangular-shaped hands with knobbly fingers are said to represent a philosophical nature. Cone-shaped hands with long thin and tapering fingers show artistic ability. Short spade-like hands are practical by nature. Narrow handed people with pointed fingers are thought to be psychic.

The nails if bitten show nervousness. White flecks show a lack of minerals (particularly zinc). Ridges running across them indicate a serious or severe illness which has affected growth.

In looking at the hand, account is made of the length of the fingers, the presence of the humps on the palms (referred to as mounts), the shape of the skin creases, and the positions and shapes of the lines on the palm.

Figure 8 shows the mounts and the main lines on the hand and the wrist.

The Life Line – this shows the energy of the individual. A broken line does not mean death, but there may be health problems at that point in life. The timing is worked out according to the proportions of the broken parts of the line.

The Line of the Head – this shows the mental capacities of the individual. If it is very close to the Line of the Heart, it indicates that the individual will be ruled by the head not the heart. The deeper and better formed it is, supposedly the clearer in mind is the individual. Also, they are less liable to disorders of the brain.

The Line of the Heart – this is to do with the emotions, attractions, romance and moods. The deeper, clearer and more continuous it is, supposedly the stronger is the individual's heart.

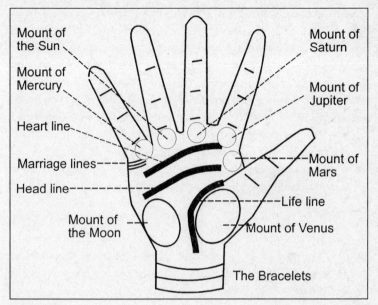

Mount of
the Sun

Mount of
Mercury

Heart line

Marriage lines

Head line

Mount of
the Moon

Mount of
Saturn

Mount of
Jupiter

Mount of
Mars

Life line

Mount of Venus

The Bracelets

Figure 8

The Bracelets – the more there are, supposedly the longer will one live. If the first ring rises onto the palm itself it indicates an internal organ problem. If the second one also arches towards the palm then it can indicate bladder problems or period problems in women.

The Marriage Lines – these apparently indicate the number of serious relationships (marriages or affairs) an individual might have.

Chains or garland-like marks near lines are thought to have significance. Chains near the Line of the Head are thought to be indicative of a tendency to migraine. Chains or breaks on the Line of the Heart might indicate circulatory problems.

The Mounts are not always easy to discern, basically because they are often mistaken for the pads of the palms. When you look along the flat of the palm you will see three pads on the palm between the fingers. The Mounts are on either side. A well developed Mount of Jupiter makes the individual very daring, while lines on it may indicate accidents if one is not careful. A well developed Mount of Saturn may make the individual morose by nature, with markings on it indicating potential problems with nerves. A well developed Mount of the Sun is a fortunate sign, but markings may indicate misfortune. A well developed Mount of Mercury makes the individual a good communicator, while markings may indicate potential problems with the voice and throat. A well developed Mount of the Moon may indicate a nervous temperament. Markings on it may indicate a tendency to react to the phases of the Moon. A well-developed Mount of Venus is thought to be a blessing, although markings may indicate problems with one's self image leading to eating disorders or stimulant abuse.

As with the section on Astrology, professional Palmists might disagree with the interpretations given, so I must repeat that these are common beliefs in Folk Medicine as they have been told to me.

Pendulum Dowsing

The Ancient Roman Augurs practised the art of *Dactylomancy*, or dowsing with finger rings. It is a practice which has survived to the present day and developed into the branch of complementary medicine known as *Radiesthesia*.

Essentially, a weight (a ring or some such object) is suspended on a thread then held over a specimen (a hair, or spot of saliva, blood or urine) from an individual while a question is mentally asked. The way the pendulum swings gives the dowser or radiesthetist the answer.

This method is commonly used in Folk Medicine to predict the sex of a baby before it is born. Some dowsers are incredibly accurate, scoring virtually one hundred per cent success.

The pattern of swing answer is very much an individual thing. Some people get a circular clockwise movement for a 'yes' response, an anti-clockwise response to a 'no', and a too-and-fro oscillation for a 'don't know.' The would-be dowser must determine his/her own responses before progressing further.

Such pendulum dowsing is often used to determine whether or not a treatment, be that an orthodox medicine, herbal remedy or homoeopathic preparation, is suitable for the individual. Again, with the pendulum over the remedy (whatever it is) and the individual's specimen in the other hand, the dowser mentally asks whether the remedy will be right for the individual.

It is claimed that most people ought to be able to dowse given proper training.

Urine divination

Uroscopy, the art of using the urine to divine someone's health is another practice which dates back to antiquity. When a man was leaving home for a long period of time, it was customary to leave a specimen of his urine in a closed glass bottle or jar. If the urine became cloudy it was said to indicate that he was in trouble or ill, while if it cleared it showed that he had recovered and was well again.

Dr John Hall (1575–1635), the son-in-law of William Shakespeare and an eminent Jacobean physician left a case-book which gives us a good insight into the practice of Medicine during the seventeenth century. In his house in Stratford-Upon-Avon, Warwickshire, are facsimiles of letters which patients sent to him along with specimens of their urine, so that he could diagnose their complaints and prescribe accordingly.

I recently came across another old practice in a Yorkshire family. When a member of the household fell ill a specimen of their urine was taken and boiled. Nail clippings were then dropped in. If they floated it was said to show that the illness had not reached a peak. If they sank the recovery was just around the corner. I was actually shown this with a patient for whom I wanted to prescribe an antibiotic. The urine was prepared, the nails dropped in and I watched them sink. No antibiotic was given and the patient completely recovered within two days.

I was also told by the family guru that spitting in one's urine immediately after passing it ensured that no illness would come that day. It is interesting to note that the case notes for that individual were almost non-existent as there had only ever been a couple of doctor-patient contacts.

Chapter Four

Follow the Signs

*'Everything born of Nature is fashioned
to reveal its intrinsic properties.'*

Paracelsus

In Antiquity man searched for remedies according to three principles which were collectively known as the *Doctrine of Signatures*. First among these was the idea that plants and animals possessed distinctive markings or features which would provide a clue as to their therapeutic usefulness. Second was the belief that by observing the instinctive behaviour of ailing animals, the way they rested and the sort of foods they nibbled at, one could be led to the natural medicine for a complaint. Finally, there was the notion that wherever an illness was prevalent there would also be found a remedy source in the nearby vicinity.

Many herbs and flowers are still used in Folk Medicine today. Indeed, we can often find clues to their medical uses when we look at both the common English name and the common country or traditional names which have been applied and retained over the years. For example, when a plant is called after a part of the body, particularly if part of the word ends in 'wort', there is an implication that it was used as a remedy for some condition associated with that organ or body part. The word *'wort'* comes from the Old English *'wyrt,'* meaning *useful plant*. Thus, the *Lungwort* was perceived to be useful for lung problems. This medical use is also indicated by two of its common country names – *Oak Lungs and Lung Moss*.

The Doctrine of Signatures might sound very naive, yet for many, many centuries it was the main method by which medicines were discovered. Interestingly, the same principles seem to have been applied by different cultures across the globe.

The signs could relate to the shape of the leaves, flowers, roots, seeds or bark. Sometimes the colour of the plant or its juice would be thought significant. And sometimes, it would be its smell that led the simpler (the preparer of simples or herbal medicines) to investigate and apply the plant in the practice of his Art.

Let us now look at some of the signs that led our ancestors to find their remedies among the woods, fields and hedgerows of the countryside.

Adder's Tongue (Ophioglossum vulgatum), is a small fern with small oval leaves which has a flowering part which resembles an adder's tongue. A preparation of it was called the Green Oil of Charity, which was used for treating all sorts of bites, stings and wounds. A handful of the leaves boiled in fat or olive oil is thought to heal bruises, chilblains, ulcers and stings and bites.

Aspen and *poplar* were both once used in the treatment of feverish conditions, because their leaves 'tremble' when even a fine breeze passes over them. An infusion of the powdered bark was drunk.

Birthwort (Aristolochia longa), a herb introduced to England and once grown in monastery gardens was thought to be useful for easing the delivery of a baby, or hastening the delivery of the after-birth. It was not considered safe for pregnant women, however, since it could induce an abortion. The sign indicating its effect was the greenish-yellow flower whose shape resembled the female womb and birth canal. A mere pinch of the powdered root was given.

Burdock (Arctium lappa), also called *Love Leaves and Clot-bur*, is a distinctive plant with wavy leaves and large purple flowers which grows around old ruins. Its small burs attach themselves to passing animals, thence disseminating the plant widely. It is a useful herb for urinary problems and stones, the appearance of the burs resembling the sort of stones which form in the kidneys and pass painfully down the ureters to produce blood and clots in the urine. About a third of an ounce of the sliced root in three-quarters of a pint of water, soaked overnight provides a soothing remedy for the urinary system. It was thought to ease the spasm and hasten the passage of a stone when a glass was taken twice a day.

Calamint (Calamintha officinalis), also known as *Bruisewort*, is a green herb which grows along the banks of streams. Its green juice was thought to look like bile, hence its use in gall bladder disease and disorders of the 'spleen.' It was considered very useful for dealing with bruises if its leaves were soaked in wine then applied to the injured surface.

Castor Oil Plant (Ricinus communis), also called *Christ's Hand*, was used by the Egyptians and is described in the Ebers Papyrus of about 1550 BC. It grows in tropical, sub-tropical and temperate zones in the world. Its oil has been a valuable commodity for many centuries. Its hand-shaped leaves indicate its general healing content. The oil is useful in all sorts of skin ailments when applied directly.

Catmint (Nepeta cataria), also called *Catwort or Cat's Delight*, is well known to attract cats. It is an example of the principle of analogy, whereby the behaviour of ill animals led people to a remedy. Drinking an infusion of the leaves as a herbal tea is thought to be good for the stomach and digestion. It also induces sweating, thereby being thought to be useful in colds.

Celandine, Greater (Chelidonium majus), used to be used in jaundiced conditions, because of the bright yellow juice which was extractable from it. It was also known as *Swallow-wort, Devil's Milk and Witchwort*, indicating its use in protecting against evil spirits. It is a herb which can be poisonous internally and corrosive when applied to the skin, even although it does have a use when touched on a wart – hence yet another name – *Wartwort*.

Celandine, Lesser (Ranunculus ficaria), also known *as Pilewort*, was used as a topical remedy for varicose veins, haemorrhoids or piles, or as a general poultice. The whole herb was scalded in boiling water or oil, then applied when cool night and morning. The sign leading to its use was the shape of its knobbly roots, which resembles a collection of prolapsed haemorrhoids or piles (also colloquially known as *the fig*, hence its common name).

Couch grass (Agropyron repens), also called *Twitch grass, Dog grass, Dog tooth*, is another example of a plant that dogs and cats instinctively chew when their stomachs are upset. Culpepper says:

> *"If you know it not....watch the dogs when they are sick and they will quickly lead you to it."*

The bruised roots should be boiled in wine, then drunk in a small quantity in order to cleanse the stomach and open the bowel.

Cuckoo-pint (Arum maculatum), is a distinctive plant also known as *Lords and Ladies*. It is found in shady hedgerows in the spring and summer, its phallic-like flower giving the sign of its use as a potent aphrodisiac. The name is derived from the Anglo-Saxon *cucu*, meaning lively, and *pintle*, meaning penis. It is highly poisonous while flowering, so I mention it merely from its historic interest.

Dandelion (Taraxacum officinale), also called *Devil's milk-pail*, like the Greater Celandine was often used for jaundiced conditions because of its yellow appearance. It is well-known as a digestive aid and as a diuretic which may be of value in slimming.

Elecampane (Inula helenium), *the Wild Sunflower, or Horseheal*, was imported to England by returning crusaders. It had apparently been used by the Saracens to deal with muscular injuries and respiratory ailments of their horses. The whole herb dropped into a hot bath soothes aches and muscular pains. An inhalation of the herb in steam soothes respiratory catarrh and coughs.

Eyebright (Euphrasia officinalis), also called *Clear-eye*, is a small plant with red or purple and white flowers, spotted with yellow 'eyes'. It should never be taken internally, except in homoeopathic dilutions. A handful of the whole herb boiled in three-quarters of a pint of water makes an excellent lotion. Bathing the eyes in this lotion several times a day is excellent for eye strains and minor eye problems It was also once thought to enhance the vision.

Figwort (Scrophularia nodosa), also called the *Scrofula Plant, Brownwort, Carpenter's Herb and Poor Man's Salve*, grows in ditches and damp places. It used to be used to cure the King's Evil or Scrofula, hence one of its alternative names. Like the Lesser Celandine (Pilewort) it resembles a collection of prolapsed haemorrhoids or piles (also colloquially known as the fig, hence its common name.) The whole herb or its leaves boiled in water or oil then strained were used to treat piles, skin problems and all sorts of scratches and cuts (such as may be suffered by a carpenter.) Sometimes the leaves would also be used as a poultice.

Foxglove (Digitalis purpurea), is also known *as Witches' Gloves, Bloody Fingers and Dead Man's Thimbles* is well known as the plant from which the heart drug Digitalis and its derivative Digoxin were first prepared. It is quite poisonous, however, since the dosages needed to treat heart failure are very small and refined. The sign of its poisonous nature is beautifully encapsulated in its country names.

Garlic (Allium sativum), also known as *Gypsy's Onions*, was thought to be good for all conditions affecting 'tubes' since it has a hollow stem.

Ginger (Zingiber officinale) is a well known plant and spice, the convolutions of its rhizome resembling the appearance of the bowel. As such it is a useful aid to digestion and helps treat diarrhoea, nausea, colic and indigestion. The root can be chewed raw before meals to prevent colic. Alternatively, ginger tea and honey may be taken.

Liquorice (Glycyrrhiza glabra), is a native plant of Southern Asia and Europe. It was cultivated by the Greeks, Persians and the Romans. The monks of England knew of its stomach ulcer-healing ability and its value as a laxative. Indeed, one of the symptoms of a bleeding stomach ulcer, referred to as *melaena*, is the appearance of black bowel movements – which is precisely the effect one sees after eating a lot of liquorice, hence the signature. An infusion of the root, or grating the root with some other herbal tea works well in reducing the problems associated with a stomach ulcer.

Liverwort (Anemone hepatica), this herb originates from temperate Northern zones. Its lobulated leaves were thought to resemble the structure of the liver. It should be noted that there is also an *English Liverwort* (Peltigera canina), which is actually a greyish lichen seen on old dykes and walls. It too is thought to have been useful in liver diseases when taken in an infusion. It was also considered to be effective against rabies.

Lungwort (Sticta pulmonaria), also called *Oak Lungs and Lung Moss*, grows in woods and thickets. Its spotted leaves resemble lungs, hence the belief that it was useful in lung and respiratory problems. A teaspoonful of the dried herb in a cup of water, three times daily, is said to relieve catarrh and bronchial congestion.

Nettle (Urtica urens), the *Common Stinging Nettle,* also called *Sting-leaf* and *Bad Man's Plaything* is useful as a lotion prepared from the whole plant in all burning or stinging skin conditions. Hence, the nature of the irritation it produced was its signature. A handful of the whole herb or its leaves boiled in water then cooled makes a useful lotion for such conditions and for easing the pain of small superficial burns.

Nutmeg (Myristica fragans), was thought to be effective in all mental and brain disorders because of the resemblance of the nutmeg to the surface of the brain. Also, its intoxicating fragrance was believed to reinforce its potential use in conditions where the mind seemed intoxicated. For the same reason it was thought to be an effective hypnotic or sleep-inducer when grated and sprinkled in a milk drink at night.

Plantain (Plantago major), commonly grows on waste ground. It is also known as *Snakeweed, Englishman's foot and St. Patrick's Leaf*. It used to be used as an amulet, a leaf kept in the pocket while on the moors being considered a protection against snake-bite. Its long flat ribbed leaves were considered a sign that it could be used to treat ailments associated with the hands, feet, the fingers or the nerves. The ground up leaves boiled in water or oil then allowed to cool, make a soothing lotion for infections and inflammations of the hands and feet. Alternatively, the leaves as a poultice could be used.

Pumpkin (Cucurbita maxima), also called *Wormseed*. For centuries the seeds of the pumpkin have been used to expel worms from the body. The sign is that the pumpkin seed resembles the segmented body of a tapeworm. The seeds should be sun-dried, then a tablespoon of them should be crushed in a tablespoon of castor oil and a tablespoon of honey. This mixture is taken after a preceding day's fast. Chewing the sun-dried seeds regularly thereafter were thought to prevent a reccurrence of the infection.

Rose (Rosacea), is an ancient remedy for the heart, the signature being the heart shape of the rose leaves. Two dessertspoonfuls of the rose petals should be crushed and mixed thoroughly with one dessertspoonful of honey. Traditionally, this was to be left outside for twenty-four hours to soak up the energies of the moon and the sun. A stock should be made (from the above quantities mixed with a pint of boiling water) and a dose taken every morning.

St John's Wort (Hypericum perforatum), also called *Holy Herb, Balm to the Warrior's Wound, Touch and Heal*. This herb in mediaeval times was thought to have been imbued with healing powers because it blooms around the time of the Saint's Day. The red juice of its curiously perforated leaves was thought to represent the blood of the saint and indicated its ability to cure wounds. An infusion of the finely chopped flowers, drunk in a tablespoon three times a day, was used to cure all types of minor haemorrhage, and to treat all manner of acute pains. Toothache, arthritis, and crushed fingers and toes are all said to respond to it. It is also used externally as the *Oil of St John's Wort*. This is made by preparing a handful of the finely chopped flowers in simmering oil. This balm is useful for all sorts of sores, ulcers and wounds.

Self-Heal (Prunella vulgaris), also called *All Heal, Sicklewort and Hookweed*. It grows close to the ground and throws out distinctive violet coloured flowers which have a distinctive spike, like a hook or a sickle – hence its signature. An infusion of its flowers, drunk in a tablespoon three times a day was thought to heal wounds, ulcers and headaches. It was also recommended for period problems and stomach disorders.

Shepherd's Purse (Capsella bursa-pastoris), also called *Shepherd's Heart and Sanguinary*, grows on the sides of roads and waste ground. Its tiny seed boxes, like Shepherd's purses, or tiny hearts, imply its use in heart and circulatory problems. It is an excellent herb for dealing with period problems and small haemorrhages. It is an excellent one for stopping recurrent nose bleeds. A handful of the herb can be chewed on its own twice a day, when there is such a problem. Alternatively, an infusion of a handful of the whole herb in three-quarters of a pint of water, infused overnight makes a good stock. A tablespoon taken two or three times a day usually has a marked effect. As an acute remedy, a cotton wool ball can be soaked in the stock solution and applied directly into a bleeding nose, often with good effect when pressure is applied externally at the same time.

Skullcap (Scutellaria galericulata), also called *Hoodwort and Helmet Flower*. This is a very famous herb which has been used for centuries. The flowers shaped like a helmet with the visor closed was thought to indicate its value in disorders of the mind and the head. An infusion of a handful of the whole herb boiled in half a pint of water is allowed to cool. A small glass twice a day is said to relax one beautifully and induce a good night's rest. Skullcap is also available in tablet form from herbalists, but at the time of writing I feel that it is a herb which should be used with great caution and not used repeatedly since there is a suspected risk of it causing liver impairment.

Strawberry (Fragaria vesca), because of the resemblance of the fruit to the shape of the heart, it was perceived to be of value in heart disorders. It is certainly a useful nerve-calmer and does seem to give energy – provided one is not allergic to it.

Walnut (Juglans nigra), a tree which produces characteristic wrinkled nuts. The nut was thought to resemble the convoluted surface of the brain, hence the nuts were considered to be valuable in disorders of the mind and of the brain. Similarly, the wrinkling was considered analogous to the ageing of the skin, so a lotion of the leaves was considered useful in dealing with skin problems like eczema, as well as for general skin care.

Willow (Salix alba), a tree that classically grows in damp places because it is a 'water-lover.' Because of this, it was believed that it would hold the answer to conditions which were rampant in damp conditions, like ague and rheumatism. It was this very idea which led the Reverend Edward Stone to discover the value of willow bark.

For some unknown reason, the clergyman tasted the bark of a willow while he was out walking one day in the summer of 1758. To his surprise he found that it tasted much the same as Peruvian Bark, the standard treatment for malaria and feverish conditions in those days. Having some knowledge of the Doctrine of Signatures he wondered whether the willow bark might also be effective. At any rate his investigations were to prove successful and to have momentous importance. Willow bark became widely used through-out Europe as a cheaper alternative to the expensive Peruvian Bark. Then, as the scientific approach continued to advance, a research race began to discover the nature of the active pain-killing and fever-cracking agent. It was to lead eventually to the discovery of one of orthodox medicine's most powerful drugs – aspirin.

And it was just one example of many which have shown that the Doctrine of Signatures held more than a kernel of truth.

Chapter Five

Vital Fluids and Vital Herbs

'Diversity of humours breadeth tumours'

Medieval Proverb

'The qualities of medicines are
considered in respect of man, not of
themselves; for those simples are called
hot which heat our bodies; for those
cold which cool them; and those
temperate which work no change at all.'

Nicholas Culpeper

When early man eventually gave up his nomadic existence as a hunter and food-gatherer, he settled on the land and began to grow crops. As he became intimately involved with the process of nurturing his crop, he would inevitably realise that three factors were necessary to grow food – heat from the sun, water and earth. One can thus easily imagine how the early settlers would deify these requisites of plant life to form a basic cosmology or theory of the universe. To these three he would add the invisible cosmic element of air, or breath in order to account for the special needs of both man and animals.

And so, we can see how a theory of the *'Elements'*, – *Earth, Air, Fire and Water* – could have developed to explain the nature of the universe. However, it would not account for the fact that plants and animals are different from the rest of the inanimate world. In order to allow for this, he would develop the concept of some form of Vital Force or energy.

Anthropology tells us that this simple philosophical blueprint has recurred across the globe throughout the centuries. It was refined by the Ancient Greeks in the fifth century BC. Hippocrates of Cos, often referred to as the Father of Medicine, developed the idea that the four Elements acted upon by the Vital Force became activated into *humours or Vital Fluids* once they had been assimilated and absorbed into the body.

There were four Vital Fluids – *Blood, Phlegm, Black bile and Yellow bile*. He taught that Air absorbed through the lungs would be transformed into Blood; Water would eventually become Phlegm; Earth (from the substance of food) would become Black Bile; and Heat or Fire would become Yellow Bile.

Aristotle added to this theory the idea of the Elements being linked to the *Four Qualities of Hot, Dry, Cold and Wet*. Each Element was conceived as being a mixture of two paired Qualities. This postulate allowed for the transformation of one Element into another, if the predominance of one quality was altered. For example, Fire which is Hot and Dry, plus Water which is Cold and Wet, could respectively lose Dryness and Coldness to form Earth, which is Cold and Dry; and Air which is Wet and Hot.

The second Century physician, Claudius Galen, further refined this theory by linking the Vital Fluids (or humours) and Qualities with the tissues of the body. From this arose the further idea that the Vital Fluids could be linked to the Temperaments of Man. There were thought to be four basic temperaments – sanguine, phleg-matic, melancholic and choleric. In addition, because these were also associated with paired qualities, a predominance of one of the pairs would result in a further four sub-types, as well as one which would be a perfect balance of all four qualities. Hence, nine constitutional types of people or nine temperaments were recognised. (Figure 9)

The pure Choleric temperament is generally confident, irascible, touchy and proud. Amition is usually well developed and there may be arrogance. The Phlegmatic, or lymphatic temperament is fussy, a bit obsessional, practical, but hates the limelight. The Sanguine temperament is excitable, impressionable, impulsive and

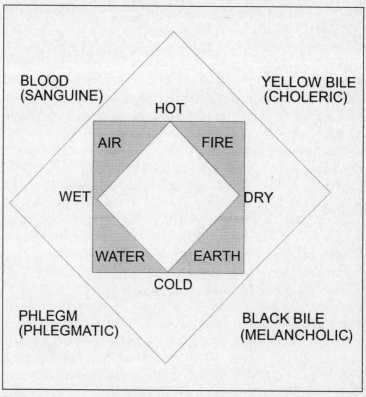

BLOOD
(SANGUINE)

YELLOW BILE
(CHOLERIC)

HOT

AIR   FIRE

WET   DRY

WATER   EARTH

COLD

PHLEGM
(PHLEGMATIC)

BLACK BILE
(MELANCHOLIC)

Figure 9

sometimes unreliable. He can sometimes seem frivolous and thoughtless to others. The Melancholic temperament is cautious, serious, industrious and solitary. There is, of course, a tendency to become depressed.

It also came to be believed that different organs were influenced by one of three *Essences or Spirits.* The heart was thought to be the site of the *Vital Spirit,* which was responsible for hope, humanity, morality, and courage. The Liver was thought of as the site of *Natural Spirit,* which nourished the body. Finally, the brain was associated with *Animal Spirit,* which gave the individual imagination, judgement and memory.

Astrological influences were also considered important, as mentioned in the chapter on medical divination. Both the Vital

Fluids and the Essences were thought to be influenced by both the Zodiacal signs and the planets.

Vital Spirit, which was responsible for one's general outlook on life was ruled by the Sun, equating pretty well with an individual's Sun sign at birth. Animal Spirit, being to do with mental processes was associated with Mercury, the swift, witty and intellectual messenger of the gods. Natural Spirit came under the dominion of Jupiter, which also ruled the action of the blood.

The Choleric temperament, which moved men to acts of valour was associated with the planet Mars. Phlegmatic, or lymphatic types were ruled by the Moon and Venus. Melancholiacs had Saturn, the 'grave councillor of the whole body,' while Sanguine people were again ruled by Jupiter.

Health was thus considered to be dependent upon a balance between the Vital Fluids, disease being the inevitable consequence of any imbalance. Treatment involved restoring the balance by reducing the *peccant* or disease-producing humour. For example, if blood was conceived to be the offending humour, then blood-letting would restore the balance. Our word *exsanguinate,* meaning to drain of blood, can be seen to originate from such practice. Similarly, *cholagogues*, remedies which affected the flow of bile; *emetics*, which caused vomiting; and *purgatives* which cleared out the bowel, were all used to remove other excessive peccant humours.

Another method of restoring balance was by utilising the *Doctrine of Contraries*. This meant that a predominantly *Moist* disease could be cured by administering a *Dry* remedy, whereas a *Hot Drug* would be most effective against a *Cold disease.* This system of pharmacology became known as *Galenism,* after the physician Galen, and the drugs came to be known as *Galenicals*.

Many Galenicals were extremely complicated, consisting of numerous ingredients of dubious value. Galen himself frequently prescribed remedies consisting of as many as one hundred ingredients. The substances used ranged from the magico-medical (pulversied Egyptian mummy foot), to the exotic (ground unicorn or rhinoceros horn), to the commonplace plants and herbs. Indeed, in our expression 'as cool as a cucumber' we see a reference to the use of this simple vegetable as a Galenical. It is a cooling agent which has been found to have a scientific rationale, since it is rich in salicylates, which are of course related to aspirin.

Blood and Urine

Since blood was the most obvious Vital Fluid, it is not surprising that its importance should have become pre-eminent in Folk Medicine around the world. Indeed, its significance is apparent in expressions such as 'life-blood', 'precious fluid', ' life-fluid', all of which have drifted into common parlance. Similarly, 'blood is thicker than water' refers to the idea of it being important in relatives, while 'hot-blooded' and 'cold-blooded,' implies a connection with the emotions.

Ancient magico-medical practices in different parts of the world led people to believe that by drinking blood one could absorb the qualities of the donor. This practice may well have derived from cannibalistic rituals of more primitive times. Drinking the blood of animals also had magico-medical significance, in that the attributes of the creature were thought to be absorbed, thereby countering the illness suffered from. For example, drinking bull's blood would give strength; hare's blood would give breath for chest problems; goat's blood would cure digestive problems, because goats seemingly have an ability to digest anything.

Blood-letting was a recognised treatment extending from the days of Ancient Egypt right down to recent times. It was performed by opening veins or by the application of leeches (which are, incidentally, being reintroduced into modern Western medical practice!) The great physician Galen advocated that blood should only be taken when the moon was waxing, or when a favourable Aspect existed between it and Jupiter. This became a fixed principle down through most of the next two millenia, as can be seen from Shakespeare's reference to it in one of his histories:

> ..Our doctors say this is no month to bleed.
> Good Uncle, let this end where it begun;
>
> Richard ll, Act 1, Scene 1

The practice continued for three more centuries then drifted into Folk Medical practice after the technique was discontinued by the medical profession.

Urine, while not being one of the four Vital Fluids often became linked with the humours in the popular mind. Since it is the fluid which is daily removed from the body, it understandably became the subject of much interest. *Uroscopy*, the art of diagnosis by looking at the patient's urine became a standard part of medical practice, as mentioned in chapter 3. Once again, William Shakespeare refers to it and the practice of purging in one of Macbeth's speeches when a doctor is summoned to cure the Lady Macbeth of her madness:

> ...*Doctor, the thanes fly from me.*
> *Come, sir, dispatch. If thou couldst, doctor, cast*
> *The Water of my land, find her disease*
> *And purge it to a sound and pristine health*

> *Macbeth, Act V, Scene lll*

Apart from being considered of value in diagnosis, the urine was thought to have curative powers of its own. The theory was that the body modified toxins and poisons, expelling them in the urine where they were immediately available to be used in treatment. Let me cite some old Scottish Folk remedies.

Deafness and tinnitus (ringing in the ears) were thought to be curable by washing the ears and instilling warm urine into them for a few moments.

Jaundice, which often produces a yellow and very dark urine, was thought to be treatable by fasting for nine days and drinking every drop of urine which one passed.

Chapped hands and sores were thought to heal up swiftly if one passed one's urine over them every morning and night.

Infected wounds were thought to be cured by applying linen soaked in the previous days urine.

Leg ulcers were similarly thought to heal when padded with urine-soaked dressings.

Dropsy (swelling of the legs, most often from congestive cardiac failure, or heart failure) was thought to respond to fasting and drinking only ones's urine for nine days, the same as one did for jaundice.

Arthritis and rheumatism was frequently treated by the application of warm urine to the affected joints and by the taking of a cup of urine night and morning.

Humoral Theories around the world

The humoral theory as outlined above was the dominant theory of Medicine in the West until the Rennaissance, when the birth of the scientific approach seemingly made a nonsense of the concepts of Hot, Cold, Moist and Dry conditions. One of the main advocates of the new approach was Santorio Santorio, a friend and contemporary of Galileo, who demonstarted that the temperature of a Hot predominent individual and a Cold predominant person was likely to be the same.

This idea that Hot and Cold was to do with temperature was a misconception, however. The concepts of Hot and Cold should really have been regarded as metaphorical terms. Indeed, this is precisely how they have been regarded in the cultures which still extensively practice medicine based upon a humoral theory.

Traditional Chinese Medicine is not strictly speaking a humoral theory, but it is based upon an Elemental Theory – the Law of Five Elements. Graeco-Arabian Medicine, the system which was Western Medicine until the Rennaissance, is still practiced throughout Asia as Unani. Indeed, the texts of Hippocrates and Galen are still quoted in this system which serves the medical needs of millions of people in the world today. Finally, Ayurvedic medicine, another humoral system is practiced throughout India in a form which has survived intact for some three thousand years.

Philologists have looked at the roots of these three quite different systems, which respectively are based upon five, four and three principles or Humour equivalents, and concluded that although there are differences in the systems yet they probably derive from a similar cosmology, or theory of the universe. As I implied earlier, the basic philosophical blueprint for the early medical systems is probably inevitable based upon observation of nature.

Folk Medicine gradually assimilates and simplifies theories. Humoral concepts still exist in the way people think about health and disease. The Hot and Cold Model is perhaps the oldest example of this. It is based upon the idea of health as a state of balance between the two opposing principles of Hot and Cold. It is still widely adhered to by Folk practitioners in rural Africa, Latin America, and by much of the population in the Western world.

In this context Hot and Cold are not thought of as temperatures, but as the effects attributable to qualities within all substances whether they be animal, vegetable or mineral. They refer to the duality of the universe, an equilibrium between the opposing dynamic forces. Health is a balance, while disease is imbalance brought about through an excess of Hot or Cold. Treatment is aimed at restoring that balance by utilising opposing principles.

Within this concept it is thought that a person can be affected by Hot and Cold either internally or externally. Internally implies the taking into the body food or drink which is excessively Hot or Cold. Externally, on the other hand occurs as the result of physical activity or exposure to the elements.

All internal factors, eg, foods and drinks are classified according to their qualities of Hot and Cold. Merely taking an excess of one or the other would not necessarily be thought to provoke an illness. If Hot was taken at an inappropriate time, however, such as when the Sun was at its zenith, then a fever might result. Similarly, taking an excess amount of Cold when the temperature was falling would be thought to result in general malaise.

External factors such as exposure to Cold winds when the body is hot and attempting to lose heat by sweating, possibly after exertion, could be conceived as the right conditions for the development of a common cold or a chill.

Treatment according to a Hot and Cold theory would necessitate an alteration in life-style, dietary modification and possibly the administration of herbal remedies according to their qualities of Hot and Cold. A clear example of this is the Folk belief that one should '*feed a fever and starve a cold.*' A fever is thought of as a condition of Hot, which must be treated by external cooling and fasting; as opposed to a cold which is a Cold illness, treated by Hot drinks, food and Hot remedies.

The spread of herbal remedies

Herbal Medicine has been practiced since the beginning of time. The discovery of the mortal remains of early neolithic shamen have demonstrated that herbs were methodically gathered and stored for probable use as medicines. It was the basis of medical practice throughout Europe until the Rennaissance when it was all but driven underground. Its ultimate development is an interesting study in history, since it parallels the settlement of America by early pioneers and the incorporation of American Indian herbal lore into the practice of what was essentially 'Frontier Medicine.'

The days of the Wild West have been captured forever in legend, books and films. A main character in this epoch, where qualified physicians were few and very far between, was the travelling medicine man, often referred to as the 'white Indian doctor.' Many of these characters were undoubted charlatans, out to make a fast buck by peddling some worthless tonic or panacea. One who was no charlatan, however, was Samuel Thomson (1769–1843), a self-educated farm boy who learned his herbalism from a local wise woman who was skilled in Frontier Medicine.

Thomson was wise enough to put his method down on paper in a book which was to become an incredible success. It was decidedly based upon the old humoral theories and the temperaments of herbs and plants. It rapidly spead Westwards, a companion to the Bible in the covered wagon-trains carrying settlers across the great continent.

Unfortunately, *physiomedicalism*, as the Thomson method became known, met considerable resistance from the rapidly developing American Medical Association towards the end of the nineteenth century. It may even have died out completely had it not been taken back to its roots by emigrants to Britain and Europe. It was a time when the soil was fertile, for the Industrial Revolution had created many great cities where people from the country had been forced to move to gain employment. The new herbalists readily found a market for their skills, since the former country people craved for their old country treatments rather than the expensive new drugs of the orthodox medical profession. Herbalism experienced a renewed popularity, to the extent that the Thomsonian approach was adopted as the basic philosophy of the fledgling organisation, the National Association of Medical Herbalists.

In this fascinating little cycle of medical history we see how orthodox medicine drove the humoral theory into the realm of Folk practice. That Folk practice travelled across the sea with the early American pioneers where it became amalgamated with the Folk practices of the American Indians. In time the Folk Medicine practices became lifted out of the pool by Samuel Thomson and formulated into a system of medical herbalism. Again, forced underground by antipathy from the American establishment, it found its way back to Europe where it flourished before being upstaged and modifiedby later herbalist theories.

Hot and Cold Herbs

Folk Medicine, being the collecting pool of knowledge for most practices which have at one time or another been established practice, tends to simplify theories, blur the edges and lose sight of origins. Herbal remedies used in Folk Medicine in Britain range from ones based upon the ancient Doctrine of Signatures to 'newer ones' which seem to have dropped into the Folk Medicine pool by followers of herbal masters like Culpeper and Thomson.

The Hot and Cold model can be clearly seen in the selection of herbs. Hot conditions characterised by fever, a sensation of being hot, flushing, swelling and redness, basically conditions of 'excess' are thought to be best dealt with by herbs which are Cold or Cooling in nature or temperament.

Cold conditions, by contrast, those characterised by feeling cold, stagnation, congestion and general slowing of processes are thought to be best dealt with by herbs which are Hot or Warming in nature or temperament.

WARMING HERBS FOR COLD PROBLEMS

Such herbs can be thought of as ones which enhance the flow of blood, thereby opening up blood vessels and improving the circulation to raise 'heat.' The sort of conditions they are used in are:–

Skin disorders – the ones thought to be due to poor cirulation and sluggishness, whereby the skin does not get enough nourishment. Also, if the circulation is less than adequate, there may be a build up in toxic-end products of metabolism, which further deplete the circulation.

Catarrhal disorders – the ones thought to be due to congested mucous membranes and sluggish circulation.

Circulatory disorders – ranging from central ones affecting the heart to produce cardiac failure; to general ones causing high blood pressure; to peripheral ones causing claudication (painful legs on walking), cold hands and feet, chilblains, varicose veins and haemorrhoids.

Arthritic and rheumatic disorders – are traditionally considered to be Cold disorders which necessitate warming or hot remedies to ease pain and improve mobility. The preparations might be taken by mouth or, when appropriate used topically as an ointment or embrocation.

The following herbs are considered to be Warming (you will note that some of them have already been mentioned in chapter 4, since their indications had been indicated through the Doctrine of Signatures). Herbalists today would consider that they work through a circulatory stimulation mechanism, either central or peripheral in action:–

Betony, cayenne, cinnamon, elecampane, fennel, feverfew, figwort, garlic, hawthorn, horse-radish, hyssop, mustard, nettle, peppermint, sage, yarrow.

Betony (Stachys Betonica), also called *Bishopswort, Wood Betony and Sentinel of the Woods,* a few leaves infused as a tea, drunk twice a day is considered useful for catarrhal headaches, sinusitis and muzzy-headedness.

Cayenne pepper (Capsicum annum) is used as a tonic for the heart, for aching legs and sluggish circulation, to enhance fertility and for arthritis. About a quarter of a teaspoon is taken in a cup of water twice a day for as long as felt necessary. Once improvement occurs, the treatment is stopped.

Cinnamon (Cinnamonum zeylanicum) is used for stimulating the digestive system when there is thought to be sluggishness. It stimulates bowel movement and is also useful for sluggish lower limb circulation, difficulty clearing catarrh and for relieving nausea. It is taken like cayenne for as long as felt necessary.

Elecampane (Inula helenium), also called *Wild Sunflower* and *Horseheal,* is useful for respiratory catarrh and for clearing up bronchitis when taken as a herbal tea.

Fennel (Foeniculum vulgara), is useful for settling constipation, for enhancing fertility and for helping rheumatism. It is also reputed to be helpful in dealing with obesity. The leaves can be chewed.

Feverfew (Chrysanthemum parthenium), also called *Nosebleed*, is useful for sluggish periods in women, painful periods, arthritis and migraine. The flowers made into an infusion and taken as a herbal tea are beneficial twice a day. Also, if the leaves are made into a poultice then they are said to be useful for relieving painful, swollen joints.

Figwort (Scrophularia nodosa), also called *the Scrophula Plant, Brownwort, Carpenter's Herb and Poor Man's Salve,* is used as an ointment for skin problems, including eczema, wounds and sores, and haemorrhoids. The whole herb or leaves boiled in water or oil, made a useful mode of treatment. Alternatively, the soaked leaves can be used as a poultice.

Garlic (Allium sativum), also known as *Gypsy's Onions*, is good for the circulatory system and blood pressure. A whole clove chewed daily, or proprietory garlic pills can be taken. Parsley is worth chewing afterwards in order to counter the characteristic pungent garlic odour.

Hawthorn (Crataegus monogynova), also *called Hagthorn, i*s generally considered tonic to the heart and circulatory system. The leaf buds when chewed taste like *Pepper and Salt*, yet another country name. A poultice made out of the leaves is good for drawing boils and splinters which have been slow to form or come out.

Horse-radish (Cochlearia armoracia), is used as a remedy to stimulate the appetite, expel woms and parasites and relieve urinary tract infections. One or two roots, grated down and taken daily in several divided doses before meals. Taking bread at the same time will reduce the heat in one's mouth.

Hyssop (Hyssopus officinalis), is used as an expectorant for troublesome respiratory catarrh. An infusion of the flowers as a herbal tea twice or three times a day is recommended. It is also well known as a *diaphoretic,* which is a preparation which induces sweating during an infection.

Mustard (Sinapsis alba), also called *Gold Dust,* can clear catarrh and bronchitis when a weak infusion is sipped sparingly throughout the day. Too much, however, and it will overheat the stomach and induce nausea.

Nettle (Urtica urens), the *Common Stinging Nettle*, also called *Bad Man's Plaything*, and *Sting-leaf,* makes a useful lotion for burns and all stinging and itching conditions of the skin. A handful of the whole herb should be boiled in water. An infusion taken as a herbal tea is also well known as a useful treatment for arthritis and rheumatism.

Peppermint (Mentha piperita), is a well known general tonic. An infusion as a herbal tea is good for relieving congested headaches, stimulating the stomach and easing the pain of varicose veins.

Rose (Rosacea), an ancient remedy for the heart (see Chapter 4). Traditionally, two dessertspoonfuls of the crushed petals should be mixed with a dessertspoonful of honey and taken every morning. The old-timers say that it should be left out of doors for twenty-four hours to absorb the energies of the moon and the sun.

Sage (Salvia officinalis), taken like hyssop is a powerful diaphoretic. Gargling with an infusion of the leaves eases a sore throat and hastens the passage of catarrh. A sage bath is also an excellent restorative for aching muscles and joints. A footbath quickly eases the footsore walker.

Yarrow (Acillea millefolium), also called *Bloodwort, Woundwort and Staunch-weed,* is another diaphoretic. Its reputation as a wound healer and herb which reduces haemmorhage goes back many centuries. It is well known as a herb which is good for easing sluggish and irregular periods, easing period pains and for stimulating the appetite.

COOLING HERBS FOR HOT PROBLEMS
These herbs are generally good for slowing down or relaxing processes in the body. They are used when there are inflammations with feelings of heat, burning, etc.

Digestive disorders – where there is inflammation of the stomach or intestines, loss of appetite and pain. These remedies are considered as *bitters* by modern herbalists.

Spasm problems – where muscles, intestines or internal tubes go into acute spasm to produce cramp pains. This is a common mechanism of pain, seen in Irritable bowel syndrome, dyspepsia, some forms of constipation and migraine. These remedies are considered as relaxants by modern herbalists.

Overactivity problems – where nervous activity seems to produce symptoms of unease. This includes anxiety states, tension headaches, insomnia.

The following herbs are considered to be Cooling:–

Chamomile, dandelion, gentian, hops, self-heal, skullcap, valerian, wormwood, yellow dock,

Chamomile (Anthemis nobilis), was known to the Ancient Egyptians as a cure for ague. They dedicated it to their Gods Thoth and Imhotep. It is an excellent relaxant and sedative which can ease the spasms of irritable bowel syndrome, nocturnal cramps, period pains and nervous irritability. Beatrix Potter may have done much to broadcast its use as a sleep-inducer when she had Mrs Rabbit send her errant child Peter Rabbit off to bed with a large spoon of Chamomile tea. An infusion of the flowers makes a bitter herbal tea which is made palatable with spearmint, honey or grated liquorice root.

Dandelion (Taraxicum officinale), also called *Devil's Milk-Pa*il, is a well known bitter which has been used for digestive problems for centuries, as a laxative, diuretic and aid to slimming. The leaves can be freely chewed, although over-indulgence can cause nausea. An infusion of the leaves taken as a herbal tea is also quite a useful way of taking the herb. As yet another alternative, the dried roots, ground and powdered can make a coffee substitute.

Gentian (Gentiana lutea), is a well known bitter, useful for digestive troubles and as an anti-inflammatory remedy. It is useful for easing nausea. It also works as a calming agent in anxiety states. Stock can be made by infusing an ounce of the grated root in a pint of boiling water. Two tablespoonfuls three times a day is the usual dosage when needed.

Hops (Humulus lupulus), is a calming, sedative, bitter. It eases digestive inflammations and calms the mood. It is taken as a herbal tea and is almost a specific hangover remedy.

Self-Heal (Prunella vulgaris), also called *All Heal, Sicklewort and Hookweed*. An infusion of its flowers, drunk by the tablespoon three times a day seems to promote healing of wounds, ulcers (internal and external) and headaches. It also relieves period and irritable bowel cramps.

Skullcap (Scutellaria galericulata), also called *Hoodwort and Helmet Flower*. An infusion of a handful of the whole herb in half a pint of water is allowed to cool. A small glass twice a day is an excellent relaxant and promoter of sleep. It is also available from herbalists in tablet form. It should, however, be used with great caution, preferably under the supervision of a doctor or herbalist, since there is a suspected risk of it causing liver impairment.

Valerian (Valeriana officinalis), also called *All Heal* (so do not confuse with Self-Heal above!), *St George's Herb and Garden Heliotrope*. This is another wonderful relaxant and sleep-inducer. Unfortunately, since it too may have a dubious effect upon the liver, it should only be taken under the supervision of a doctor or herbalist.

Wormwood (Artemisia absinthium), also called *Green Ginger*. This is possibly the bitterest of all plants. Its use is summed up in the writings of Tusser (1577) in July's Husbandry:

> *While Wormwood hath seed get a handful or twaine*
> *To save against March, to make flea to refraine:*
> *Where chamber is sweeped and Wormwood is strowne,*
> *What saver is better (if physick be true)*
> *For places infected than Wormwood and Rue?*
> *It is a comfort for harte and the braine,*
> *And therefore to have it is not in vaine.*

Wormwood was used in the country to keep away fleas, insects and moths. It was strewn around the room and also put in drawers with lavendar to kill off any moths.

It was also used as an infusion as a relaxant and bitter, and as an ingredient in love potions. It is another herb which should only be taken under the supervision of a doctor or herbalist.

Yellow dock (Rumex crispus), taken as an infusion of the grated root (a teaspoon to a pint of boiling water), in a dose of one tablespoon twice a day, is good for digestive inflammations. It works well as a laxative.

Chapter Six

Airs, Waters and Places

*'Water, air, and cleanliness are the
chief articles in my pharmacopoeia.'*

Napoleon

*'When a physician moves to a new city
it is his first duty to understand the air,
water and place.'*

Hippocrates

The operating theatre was hot and humid despite the huge fan. Perspiration trickled down my forehead into my eyes so that I had to blink hard to get rid of the momentary blurring of vision. My mask clung to my face and I felt as if I would have to peel my operating gown from my body. My arms ached from pulling on the heavy retractors as I endeavoured to provide the Professor of Surgery with the best possible view of the operation site.

I had been working at the Government Fever Hospital in Hyderabad for a little over two months when the patient, a girl of about sixteen or seventeen was brought in from one of the outlying villages. By that time I had seen numerous cases of Typhoid, so the underlying diagnosis was never in doubt. Unfortunately, she had a dire complication. Her small bowel had perforated. Her condition was so weakened that there had been considerable debate about the wisdom of transferring her to the surgical unit at the Osmania Hospital. Yet it was her only realistic chance.

The Professor had operated swiftly and brilliantly. I had assisted at emergency operations in Scotland, yet never upon patients who needed surgical intervention so dramatically.

As he inserted the last stitch in the intestine and exerted traction upon the catgut suture so that I could reach down and snip with the fine scissors, he winked at me over the top of his mask. "And all because of dirty water drinking," he said.

Behind him, a huge suction bottle was full of several litres of green fluid, all of which had been oozing from the perforation in the girl's intestine into her abdominal cavity.

Her's had been a classic case. In the first week she had developed a fever. In the second week she noticed a rash (described in text books as being like 'rose spots', although in practice they are hardly ever like this), and started with diarrhoea. In the third week she became more and more ill until she developed the severe abdominal pain. This was due to the sudden bursting of an ulcer near the end of her small intestine.

The cause of Typhoid Fever is usually a bacterium called *Salmonella typhi*. It is transmitted by contamination of food or water. It is, therefore, a condition directly related to the state of food production, sanitation and water supply.

I am pleased to say that our patient made a complete recovery over the next few weeks. She had literally been hauled back from the jaws of death, since her chances of survival must have been as low as one in a hundred when she was first brought into hospital.

And as the Professor said, all because she had drunk contaminated water.

Airs, Waters and Places

Hippocrates is credited as being the first physician to have written about public health as we know it. He taught his students that they should make it their business to know about the type of water supply, the trades and occupations of the people, the type of climate and the illnesses which the local populations were subject to. By doing this, they would develop an insight into the psychological and physical development of their patients. Not only that, but by having an awareness of illness proneness of a locality, they would be in a position to devise the appropriate treatments.

Water is, of course, a fundamental requirement of life. Its purity has been recognised as being important for health for many centuries. According to Herodotus, the Ancient Greek traveller and historian, the Emperor of the Persians drank only boiled water when travelling. Large quantities were carried in silver vessels.

The act of boiling water does kill off many potential disease-producing agents. Indeed, the rural Chinese may have avoided many major water-borne epidemics over the centuries, because of their universal and traditional habit of drinking tea.

The reason why water could cause disease was not known until the nineteenth century when the science of bacteriology started identifying the microbial jungle which lurks beyond the limits of man's naked eye. It was really only then that men could effectively prevent the epidemics of conditions like Typhoid and Cholera

For centuries climate has also been recognised as having an effect upon people's well-being. People have always been aware of how damp climates and localities produce an increase in rheumatic disorders and respiratory diseases. Similarly, some areas and climates seem to be associated with gastric complaints and others with neurological or nervous states.

As medicine advanced, physicians made it part of their business to know all about waters, airs and places. Indeed, up until the last war part of the treatment which patients might be recommended could be a holiday in a particular resort to take the air or the waters. But interestingly, many of these resorts had a history extending back many centuries to the pre-Christian era.

Healing Wells

Even before the Romans came to Britain in 43 AD the Celts had established shrines and centres of healing at various wells and springs. The Romans, with their building and engineering expertise often upgraded these wells and absorbed them into their system of veneration, since their pantheon of divinities included many who looked after springs, wells and rivers. Then as Christianity spread across the land many of these Romano-Celtic wells were blessed and became accepted as valid places of pilgrimage. Indeed, in Scotland there are about two dozen wells named after St Ninian and St Columba. Churches were often built in the immediate vicinity, since it was politically easier to absorb the older pagan beliefs rather than try to suppress them.

Over the centuries these wells became famous for their healing waters. Eye disorders, asthma, consumption, skin problems, and nervous illnesses, all of them were said to improve if one made a pilgrimage to a well and performed the well-tried ritual. Some sort of offering was often made, such as a coin – hence fostering the tradition of wishing wells. Alternatively, sometimes an article of clothing or personal item was left nearby.

In my native Scotland there are many so-called *Clootie Wells*. A clootie is a piece of cloth. When someone visits such a well they are supposed to take a piece of material (the clootie, which can be a remnant of clothing or a handkerchief, for example) soak it in the well water then dab the offending or ill part of the body with it. It is then tied to the well or hung from a nearby tree while one wishes for the illness to go away. When one leaves, one leaves the ailment behind with the clootie.

There is such a well, St Mary's Well close to the battlefield of Culloden. From Jacobite stock, my mother (who bore two sons in separate years upon the anniversary of the Battle of Culloden on 16th April, 1746) informed me that this piece of transference magic would only work for those with Scottish ancestry!

The Reformation during the sixteenth century was responsible for a change in attitude regarding the wells. Up until then people made a pilgrimage merely to sip some healing water from the well. During the Reformation there was a definite attempt to suppress such pilgrimages because they were considered idolatrous. It was then that the Medical profession took a hand.

Various doctors published pamphlets extolling the medicinal action of some of the wells, when the waters were taken in quantity. That is, when the waters were drunk regularly over a period of a week or more. The emphasis had therefore changed from the well's magico-medical power to the mineral content of the water. For example, in 1667 a certain Dr Wittie from Hull wrote about the spring water at Scarborough in Yorkshire, saying that

> *"It cleanses the stomach, opens the lungs, cures*
> *Asthma and Scurvy, purifies the blood, cures*
> *Jaunders both yellow and black, and the Leprosie."*

There were many such wells which developed a considerable reputation. Interestingly, hospitals were often built in the close vicinity in later years. As a young surgical house officer I began my career at the Bridge of Earn Hospital in Scotland, the site in earlier times of a famous well.

In other towns hydropathic (water treatment) hotels were established and the towns developed the status of Spas (after the Belgian town of Spa, which was famous for its carboniferous and chalybeate springs). All sorts of hydropathic treatments were performed there and before long it became fashionable for the rich and famous to travel to the spas to take 'the cure.'

Spas and Health Resorts

In assessing the needs of a patient, the dutiful physician of yesteryear would try to work out the deficiencies or excesses of the patient's illness and match it up with the beneficial atmosphere of a particular part of the country or of some suitable foreign resort. In doing so, the temperature, moisture content of the atmosphere, pressure and oxygen content were all taken into account.

Lung and chest complaints were thought to benefit from areas with pure air, a stable temperature, an abundance of sunshine and opportunity for mild exercise.

Tuberculosis, or consumption of the lung (as it used to be referred to) was said to respond well to a sea voyage. A recommended trip for British patients who could afford it, was to take a slow cruise to Australia, ideally beginning in October and arriving in early January. It was then suggested that some time be spent in the table-land of New South Wales, Queensland or New Zealand, but certainly not in the coastal towns, before starting the return voyage in mid-February. For those unable to tolerate such an arduous sea trip, a dry inland climate was recommended, such as Egypt or South Africa. Finally, for those unable to afford the trip abroad, then resorts on the Isle of Wight or the South coast of England were advised.

Patients suffering from chronic bronchitis with much expectoration of mucus were advised to seek a dry climate. Madeira, the Azores and the Canary Islands were considered ideal for the affluent, while those with lesser means were advised to seek the airs of English resorts such as Hastings, Ventnor and Torquay.

Asthma was (and still is) a much misunderstood condition. It was regarded as something which one contracted, like an infectious illness. If it began in a moist part of the country, then one was advised to seek a dry atmosphere. On the other hand, if it began in a dry inland place then the advice was to spend time at the sea. Resorts at high altitude were considered particularly beneficial, favoured ones being in the Pyrenees, the Alps and the Andes.

Heart conditions were thought to benefit from bracing, moderate climates. Sudden changes in temperature and humidity were to be avoided, as were high altitudes.

The Italian Lakes in the Summer were thought to be especially good.

Kidney disorders were thought to need dry and hot climates, preferably at sea level or low altitude. The belief was that in order to rest the kidneys one had to stimulate the function of the skin. Thus in a dry and hot climate the blood supply to the skin would open up, taking away ill humours which would be carried away as one visibly perspired. Cold and moist climates, on the other hand, were thought to close down the skin blood supply, thereby driving the ill humours back towards the kidneys.

Bombay, Cairo, the Cape of Good Hope and the French Riviera were all considered suitable climates. In England, the resort towns of Brighton, Folkstone and Ventnor were particularly recommended.

Digestive disorders were thought to benefit from sea air, moderate climates and plenty of exercise. Congestion of one form or another was perceived to be the problem. This was thought to be worsened by too hot a climate and too high an altitude. Accordingly, the Mediterranean shore was recommended.

As we saw above, water has always been recognised as a vital principle. We simply cannot live without water. It revives us when we are thirsty and very often just drinking clear water makes us feel better. It sometimes seems as if drinking it takes away unpleasant tastes, nausea and the feeling of unease.

The constituents of water was also thought to be of importance for health. Different areas of the country have different types of water, which seem to have had an effect upon the general health of communities. Modern epidemiological studies have confirmed this by showing that areas with a hard water supply have a lower incidence of coronary heart disease than do areas supplied with soft water. Indeed, the greatest average longevity seems to be directly associated with the hardest water supply, while very soft water areas seem to have higher rates of heart disease.

Spas and health resorts where people went (and still go) to take the waters were associated with different mineral contents. Like the climatic conditions which they boasted, they were also thought to be particularly good for certain conditions.

Taking the waters meant both bathing in and taking drinks of the spring waters. Hydropathic hotels, health farms and clinics could be found all over the world. Indeed, with a resurgence of interest in Naturopathic Medicine these centres may well find themselves restored as health resorts.

A typical day at a spa during the last century would involve rising at about 6am and walking to the spring to drink a glass of water while listening to a small orchestra. A short walk of about fifteen minutes up and down a terrace or along a promenade would be followed by another glass of water, then another walk, before taking a third glass. There would then be a walk back to the hotel and a light breakfast consisting of a roll or two and a cup of coffee or tea. The morning would be spent in leisurely pursuits before taking a bath between eleven and twelve o'clock. Lunch would be prescribed according to one's needs by a local or resident physician. After that the individual would rest to allow digestion, then take light exercise before a further course of water-drinking and promenading in the late afternoon. Light supper, again prescribed according to needs, would follow at seven to seven-thirty. Recreation or agreeable conversation was then permitted until bedtime which was no later than ten o'clock.

There is little doubt that the gentle pace of such life, the freedom from stress and a period of relative abstinence from the excesses of alcohol and rich food would benefit many people. It is a good blueprint for health, which is used in a modified form at many health farms today.

The spa waters varied considerably. Some waters were quite pleasant to take, while others demanded a certain raw self-discipline!

Indifferent Waters or simple thermal springs, are the waters which contain relatively little in the way of minerals, so that they are almost pure water. Usually they arise from warm springs and are naturally carbonated. Generally, such spas were places that people went to bathe as well as to take the waters internally. The effect of the escaping gas was thought to stimulate the skin. Often these spas were found in hilly regions.

They were thought to be especially good for nervous and excitable conditions of the nervous system and chronic skin disorders. When taken internally the waters were thought to be good for digestive and liver complaints.

British spas were found at Bath, Buxton and Matlock. European ones were Bagneres de Bigorre in the Pyrenees, Gastein in the Tyrol and Schlangenbad in the Valley of the Taunus.

Muriated Saline Waters, or simple salt waters, are waters mainly containing salt. They could be either hot or cold and most were naturally carbonated. Bathing in them was thought to stimulate the skin, thereby having a beneficial effect upon disorders of the kidneys and conditions thought to be resultant from defective kidney function, such as gout.. Drinking the waters was thought to be useful in stimulating tissue change, so that they were considered useful for people in a convalescent stage after an operation or serious illness. The amount which was drunk had to be supervised and regulated, because of the irritant effect of drinking salted water.

English spas were found at Cheltenham, Droitwich, Leamington, and Woodhall. European ones were at Baden-Baden in the Black Forest, Homburg in Taunus, Kissingen in Bavaria and Wiesbaden in Nassau.

Sulphinated Waters, or bitter waters, are waters containing Epsom or Glauber's salts (respectively hydrated forms of magnesium and sodium sulphate). Because of this chemical composition they produce a sulphur smell, a bitter taste and an aperient effect. Taken internally, these were thought to be especially good for all sluggish bowel and digestive disorders. Constipation, liver problems, gall-stones and piles were all said to improve with such treatment. Because of the aperient effect, the speeding up of the bowel movements, they were thought to hasten the metabolism, thereby exerting a slimming effect upon the obese and sufferers from rich living.

English spas were once found at Epsom (the salts were named after the original spring well in the seventeenth century), Cheltenham, Leamington, Purton and Scarborough. European ones were at Aesculap in Hungary, Birmensdorf in Switzerland and Carlsbad in Bohemia.

Sulphur Waters are waters characterised by the smell of hydrogen sulphide (rotten eggs) and other sulphurous compounds. Such waters were used both internally and externally in various types of baths. Taken internally, liver complaints, piles, catarrhal problems and the early stages of tuberculosis were all said to improve.

British spas were Harrogate in England, Moffat and Strathpeffer in Scotland, Lisdunvarna in Ireland and LLandridod in Wales. European ones were Aix-la-Chapelle, Enghien near Paris and Panticosa in Spain.

Simple Alkaline Waters, or simple soda waters, are waters mainly containing sodium bicarbonate. Because of the alkalinity of the waters these were understandably considered beneficial in countering the effects of excess acidity in the body. They were, therefore, recommended for stomach ulcers and dyspepsia, and for bladder troubles and urinary stones.

The main soda water spas were to be found on the European continent, especially at Apollinaris in the valley of the Ah, Bixin in Bohemia, Saltzbrunn in Silesia and Vacua in France.

Calcareous Waters, or lime waters, are waters which contain magnesium and calcium carbonate and sulphate. These chalky mineral waters were understandably thought to be valuable in bone deficiency conditions, like rickets, osteomalacia and osteoporosis (although the latter was not precisely diagnosed as such in those days). They were also thought to be of value for kidney and bladder stones, glandular complaints and tuberculosis. The constipating effect of the waters was rightly thought to be of value in diarrhoeal and irritable bowel complaints.

Folkestone and Scarborough were English resorts with some lime waters. Again, the main spas were to be found in Europe at Contrexeville in Vosges, Pouge in the Loire, St Galmier in the Loire and Inselbad in Westphalia.

Chalybeate Waters, or iron waters, are waters containing iron salts. Inevitably, these were all thought to be tonifying for anaemia and other disorders of the blood.

English spas with chalybeate springs were Cheltenham, Harrogate, Shelfanger in Norfolk and Tunbridge Wells. European ones were Godesberg near Bonn, Recoaro in Northern Italy and St Moritz.

NOTE Many spas on the Continent are still fully operational and health holidays can be enjoyed. For details about these, health farms and the British spas which still have facilities, one should contact your local travel agent. In addition there are several excellent Natural Medicine magazines on sale which include numerous hydropathic advertisements.

Whey and Grape Cures

At several of the higher altitude mountain spas (and some of the Scottish Hydropathic hotels) patients were often also offered whey (the fluid which runs off when cheese is made) and grape cures.

Both of these 'cures' had in fact been in use during the eighteenth century. Patients suffering from tuberculosis, chest problems and many other chronic illnesses were given these along with the mineral spa waters to cleanse their systems of toxins. Interestingly, many homoeopathic and naturopathic physicians have reinstituted these into their therapeutic repertoire for allergic and chronic illnesses.

The whey cure involved drinking warm goat's milk whey first thing in the morning an hour before breakfast. About one pint a day was the minimum, while resistant cases might be given up to four pints. It was found that the whey would produce an exacerbation of catarrh, provoking a healing crisis in people suffering from catarrhal conditions.

The grape cure involved eating between one and eight pounds of grapes a day, a proportion being taken on an empty stomach before breakfast and the rest throughout the day. Like the whey cure it will provoke a healing crisis after a few days.

Both of these treatments have waxed and waned in popularity over the last century. They are, I believe, of value in certain patients when administered under the direction of a competent health professional skilled in homoeopathic or naturopathic medicine.

Folk Medicine Baths

There are a few types of hydropathic treatment which have slipped into Folk Medicine practice. You will find references to them in the therapeutic index section of this book.

1) *Oatmeal Bath* Oat baths twice a week are very useful for very irritated skin problems. Three or four goods handfuls of oats are traditionally wrapped in a tea-towel and infused in a warm bath. Sometimes they are just dropped into the bath. The individual soaks in the bath for up to ten minutes.

2) *Epsom Baths* Sulphated waters containing Epsom salts are traditionally used for conditions like psoriasis. Two handfuls of Epsom salts in a warm bath two or three times a week will often help the psoriasis sufferer. Only a bath of ten minutes should be

used. People with heart problems are not advised to take Epsom baths.

3) Mustard Foot Bath A basin is filled with water which is hot, but not so hot that the feet cannot be immersed easily without discomfort. Into this water a tablespoonful of mustard is thrown and mixed. Ten minutes is the maximum time one leaves the feet.

4) Sitz Bath This is a bath used for all sorts of pelvic and abdominal problems, as well as for arthritic joint discomfort. It is essentially a hot hip bath which one sits upright in with the water up to the waist. The feet, however, are placed in a bucket or basin of lukewarm or cold water. There are variants of this, but this is the one which I first heard about and which I have found to be beneficial to many patients. As you will see in the therapeutic index, sometimes herbs can be added to the hot part of the bath, depending upon the problem.

Sitz baths should be taken regularly during a problem (if they are indicated) starting at a mere two or three minutes on the first day and building up to a maximum of ten minutes. For those prone to particular problems which might benefit from Sitz Baths, then two or three short Sitz Baths a week may be very beneficial.

IMPORTANT NOTE PEOPLE WITH HEART PROBLEMS SHOULD CONSULT THEIR HEALTH ADVISOR BEFORE THEY DO ANY SELF-EXPERIMENTATION WITH THEIR BATHS.

Chapter Seven

Fertility Rites and Love Charms

They told her how, upon St Agnes' Eve,
Young virgins might have visions of delight,
And soft adorings from their loves receive
Upon the honeyed middle of the night,
If ceremonies due they did aright......

The Eve of St Agnes

John Keats

Then love was the pearl of his oyster,
And Venus rose red out of wine.

The Garden of Proserpine,

Algernon C. Swinburne

In days gone-by, before the world's expanding population became a cause for concern, fertility and the ability to attract a suitor were prime considerations for people in most societies.

In early polytheistic cultures virtually everything could be explained by the intervention of a god. A list found in the tomb of Thuthmosis lll informs the reader that some seven hundred and forty gods and godesses were worshipped by the Ancient Egyptians. Inevitably, conception, pregnancy and the growth of the child until the end of breast feeding all had their own deities. The god *Khnum*, portrayed as a ram-headed god, was thought to be 'the Moulder', or the celestial potter. His function was to fashion children within the womb. In this he was assisted by *Heket,* a frog-headed goddess who actually gave life to the child as it floated in the fluid within the womb. *Taueret,* the female hippopotamis goddess looked after the woman during her pregnancy and sometimes joined with *Meskhent* at the birth of the child. This midwife goddess was represented as a woman wearing two long palm shoots on her head. It was believed that she temporarily inhabited the two birth bricks upon which Egyptian mothers crouched to give birth. Finally, *Renenet* the goddess of infant suckling presided over the feeding and suckling of the child. Every one of these deities was venerated and invoked as a matter of course during the different phases to ensure that they passed smoothly. If any were slighted then infertility, miscarriage, still-birth or drying up of milk were thought to take place.

In looking at the mythology of most early cultures we find that fertility and love deities were always particularly venerated. Yet although fertility and love are obviously related, their connection seems to be at the basic level. Fertility, in both agricultural and human terms, is important to a community because it would increase the work done, enhance efficiency and produce wealth. At least until human fertility exceeded the food supply. Love on the other hand, was important at the personal level.

The two types of deity associated with fertility and love seem to belong to different epochs in the development of a culture. The more 'primitive' the culture the more important were the fertility gods and goddesses. On the other hand, the more sophisticated and refined the culture, with the ability to sustain a large population, the greater was the liklihood of developing a pantheon of deities whose function was that of overseeing attraction, venery and love.

This seems to have been the case in Ancient Greece, where the goddess *Aphrodite* became the very essense of love. Scholars believe that she developed from an early fertility goddess to become a multiple-personality deity worshipped throughout the Ancient world.

The name Aphrodite (Venus to the Romans), was probably of oriental origin. It is likely that she was derived from the earlier Assyro-Babylonian goddess *Ishtar,* a voluptuous warrior deity, and the Syro-Phoenician goddess *Astarte*, patron deity of orgies. The spread of the various cults and the amalgamation of one into another would have been inevitable in those dim and distant days when one maritime power traded, fought and overcame another.

And so Aphrodite came to be venerated throughout the Aegean. But just as we recognise different types of love, so too was Aphrodite known by different names in different centres according to the character of the love which was being represented. Thus, *Aprodite Urania,* the celestial Aphrodite, was the goddess of pure or ideal love. *Aphrodite Genetrix* or *Nymphia,* was the protector of marriages. *Aphrodite Porne,* was the goddess of lust and the patroness of prostitutes. Finally, *Aphrodite Anosia* (the impious) was the goddess of unfaithful lovers. She was the mistress of gracious laughter, sweet deceits, the charms and delights of love.

Aphrodite spread her net wide. As Greece fell and the Roman Empire conquered its way across the world, the influence of Aphrodite lived on. As *Venus*, the goddess of love, she has inspired awe, worship and devotion right up to the present day. And almost as renowned as her was *Cupid* (known to the Greeks as Eros), a winged deity who shot invisible arrows into people which made them burn with love and passion.

There can indeed be few people today who have not heard of these two deities. At some stage in their lives they may even have tried invoking them upon their behalf!

Gods and Saints

The Folklore of Britain is intensely interesting. It is an island which has been invaded and settled by many different peoples. The Celts, Romans, Angles, Saxons, Vikings and Normans all came and conquered different parts of the country over the centuries. All of them left indelible marks on the land and inevitably contributed to the never-ending saga of oral tradition. They all brought parts of their culture, their beliefs, their Medicine.

As we saw in Chapter one, the different epochs in history have all caused a spread of ideas. Before the Romans arrived in Britain in 43 AD, the main religion was Celtic in origin. The Romans brought with them their pantheon of deities and inevitably there followed an inter-mixing of the two. Many Romano-Celtic shrines flourished across the length and breadth of the land. Then, as Christianity became the established religion throughout the Roman Empire, many of the pagan deities became absorbed into the new religion. Healing centres and popular shrines became the sites of Christian churches. And so, although Christianity on the one hand decried the ancient and pagan beliefs that had preceded it, it permitted their continued existence and reverence by adopting or identifying some of the deities with Christian saints.

The Celtic goddess *Brigid* had three aspects or personalities and was worshipped as a divinity of fertility and plenty. Her influence was wide and she was absorbed into the New Religion and identified with *St Brigid*, the patron saint of midwives, maids and newborn babies, and with *St Agnes*, the patron saint of virgins and betrothed couples. The Celtic goddess *Ceridwen,* the overseer of the mysteries of life and death became identified with *St Catherine of Alexandria.* Similarly, the goddess *Ma*, a fertility divinity originally from Asia Minor was introduced to Britain by the Romans. Some of her shrines were later to have Christian churches built upon them as she became associated with *St Mary.*

The Lover's Calendar

Special days associated with the saints were thus considered propitious times to invoke the aid of a particular saint in matters relating to fertility and love.

St Agnes' Eve on 21st January was traditionally regarded as a time for young maids to seek the saint's aid in giving them a vision of their future husband. After a day's fast the young girl had to go to bed and say a Paternoster, the Lord's Prayer in Latin, then undress while she looked heavenwards. Keeping her vision directed upwards she had to find her way to bed and lie with her hands behind her head. When sleep came, St Agnes would permit her a glimpse of her future husband. For those interested, the poem The Eve of St Agnes by John Keats recounts a tale of one young girl's attempt with this love divination invocation.

St Valentine's Day on the 14th February is known to lovers throughout the world. The actual connection with the historical St Valentine seems very tenuous. The fact is that in Roman times there was a feast called Lupercalia, which was celebrated in the middle of February.

Valentine's Day has been regarded as the main festival for love divination over the centuries. Hemp seed or rice were used together with an incantation in order to discover a future suitor. I have come across two versions which use a similar incantation. In the first a young woman made her way to a churchyard just before midnight on the eve of St Valentine. As the church clock struck midnight she took a handful of hempseed or rice and ran round the church three times, scattering the hemseed as she ran. As she did this she was supposed to repeat the words:

> *Hempseed I sow, hempseed I mow,*
> *He that will my true love be*
> *Rake this hempseed after me.*

She then had to run home, turning her head quickly as she left the churchyard gate to see a fleeting image of the future suitor, following as if to rake the fallen hempseed.

Visiting a churchyard at midnight is not to be recommended to any young girl, so the second version may have developed as a safer option. Again on St Valentine's Eve a young girl would take a large bowl of water and stand with her back to it. As she repeats the incantation she tosses a handful of hempseed or rice over her left shoulder into the bowl:

> *Hempseed I sow,*
> *Hempseed will grow.*
> *Let him who loves me*
> *Come after me and mow.*

The pattern of seeds in the water, whether they form a letter indicating a name, or a pattern indicating the profession of the unknown suitor, were divined in the same manner as tea- leaves in a cup.

Yarrow and Rosemary leaves were also used on St Valentine's Eve as a love divination. After a days fast the individual placed several yarrow and rosemary leaves upon their pillow and sprinkled them with rose water. They then retired to bed, uttering the incantation:

Sweet valentine, favour me:
In a dream let me my true love see.

During the night the future lover would appear. Not only that, but the person would know whether the relationship would last or not, according to whether the leaves had withered or not by morning.

St Mark's Eve on 24th April was used in days past to make a 'Dumb Cake', which would produce a divinatory revelation to young maids. Three maids had to jointly bake a cake late in the evening, without making a sound to each other. Then, at the stroke of midnight they each broke off a piece of cake. While they ate it they had to walk backwards towards their bedrooms (without any sound). If they were to be married, the shadow of their future husband would follow them. Either that, or a knock would come at their bedroom door in the night. If there was neither shadow nor knock, then it was presumed that the maid would always remain just that!

May Day corresponds to the Celtic feast of *Beltane*, when great fires were lit across the land. Maypoles made of birch were erected on village greens and Morris dancers performed vigorous re-enactments of ancient legends. The Green Man, Herne the Hunter, Robin Hood and Maid Marion – over the centuries all of them have been associated with the festivities of May Day.

Fertility and phallic symbolism surround this day. In Somerset, young wives wishing to become pregnant quickly used to be advised to go down to the Maypole after the revellers had retired to their beds. There she was to pull up her skirts and climb to the top of theMaypole where she would tie a garland of freshly cut flowers.

I also came across an interesting piece of Folk Medicine which I was told would guarantee that a childless couple would soon be blessed with children – if they were prepared to put their trust in the hands of the spirits of Robin Hood and Maid Marian.

A week before May Day, the couple had to go to a wood and gather nine types of greenery. The man had to cut a single branch from a healthy tree. This had to be stout enough at one end to make a longbow, and thin enough at the other to make a single arrow. At home the woman was to make an infusion of the greenery in which she was to soak articles of their underwear for two days and nights. They were then to be dried and left stained green. Over the next few days the man was to make his bow and arrow and practice until he was proficient at shooting the arrow some distance. With these preparations made, the couple were to go to their woodland before darkness fell on the Eve of May Day. Flighting the arrow, the man now seeing himself as Robin Hood, shoots his arrow as far into the undergrowth as he can. Only one shot is allowed. Together they then find the spot where the arrow landed and they wait for nightfall. As midnight approaches, they remove all of their clothes except for their 'greenwood clothes,' and they make love in their temporary roles as Robin and Marian.

Midsummer Eve and Midsummer Day were regarded as special in mediaeval times, although there is no doubt that the Summer Solstice has been celebrated since the days of the Druids and earlier. St John's Day on the 24th June was a special love divination day, since the herb St John's Wort was associated with the saint. It was said that if a sprig of this plant was worn throughout the day, then anyone who burned with desire for you would be unable to resist touching the sprig. If that sprig stayed fresh until the next day, then it was thought a sign that the love would stay fresh.

Michaelmas Day on the 29th September was another well known time when Somerset girls and boys could divine which suitor would be their best match. During the month of September they would pick crab apples and hide them in a row in some unused part of the house. Each apple was chosen to represent a person. When Michaelmas Day came the row was inspected and the most wholesome crab apple indicated the one most worthy of their love.

Halloween is notorious as being a night for witches and ghosts. It was also one of the great love divination nights. Apple bobbing was used to detect the liklihood of a strong love affair. If an apple was caught immediately then the love would be strong. If several attempts had to be made, then the love would become progressively weaker.

Another apple method was to take the pips from an apple and stick them onto one's forehead, allowing each pip to represent a suitor. The person then watched them fall off one by one in a mirror, until only one was left. It was said that the most suitable would be the one who stayed the longest.

Yet another also involved an apple and a mirror. Upon retiring to her room a maid was recommended to sit by a mirror and brush her hair by candlelight. As she ate the apple it was said that the image of a future suitor would appear behind her as a shadowy reflection.

November the first, being *All Saints Day* was regarded as a time when any of the saints could be invoked. Thus, any of the previous divinations might be thought worthy of a second attempt!

St Catherine's Day was one of the last chances for people to attempt divination for their soul-mate. This being the case, one spell involved between three and seven maids meeting on St Catherine's Day, 25th November. For the three preceeding days they each had to wear a sprig of myrtle. At eleven o'clock at night they met in a room and lit a small fire in a charcoal burner. Each cut their finger and toe-nails and tossed the pairings into the fire together with nine hairs from their head. Several herbs were added to the flames and, as the fire smouldered, the sprigs of myrtle were held in the rising fumes. Without talking, they stayed until the fire had gone out, then each made their way to bed. At midnight each one put the myrtle beneath their pillow then asked St Catherine to send an image of the future lover.

Love Charms and Potions

The use of Aphrodisiacs, (from Aphrodite, the Greek goddess of love mentioned earlier) goes back several millennia. The desire to attract a desirable mate using any method available is summed up by the expression 'all's fair in love and war.' Gaining the patronage of a goddess or saint, or using the aid of a love philtre or potion was considered to be part of that game.

It should also be noted that love potions were not only made and given to prospective suitors, or those whom one may have lusted after. In days gone-by (and even today in some countries and cultures) marriages were often arranged, so love had little to do with the process. Understandably, therefore, mothers (or even future brides themselves) might prepare love potions in order to instil love or passion into an unemotional relationship.

The Astrological associations of various herbs were considered important in Medicine. Thus, all herbs governed by the planet Venus were thought to have love potion potential. The following herbs are all *'under venus'* and have been advocated as herbal teas which might induce the feelings of Venus in the drinker:– Coltsfoot (Tussilago farfara), Marshmallow (Althaea officinalis), all the mints, Plantain (Plantago major), Thyme (Thymus vulgaris), Vervain (Verbena officinalis) and Yarrow (Achillea millefolium).

To this list of herbs are also added the following vegetables:– beans, parsnips, lentils. And the following fruits:– cherries, gooseberries and plums.

Ginseng (Panax ginseng), while not being considered a love herb, is said to be excellent for enhancing the sexual potency of both sexes.

Everyone of course knows the reputation that is enjoyed by oysters and to a lesser degree mussels, yet there are other sea foods said to aid l'amour. Eels, squid and octopus have been used throughout the Mediterranean for centuries.

Toadstones and Bezoar stones (see Chapter 2) were much sought after for inclusion in love philtres. They were pulverised and mixed with herbs of Venus and usually left outside overnight during a full moon. Some of the mixture baked in a cake or slipped into wine was thought to work extremely well.

An old Gypsy love potion was prepared from a single elecampane plant, a handful of vervain leaves and a handful of fennel and a small quantity of grated ginger. These were to be heated in an oven until they were dry and crumbly. They were then ground to a powder and a pinch of this powder, no more, was added to a flask of hot mulled wine. The couple who drank from this would experience unbridled desire.

St Albertus Magnus, or St Albert the Great, was a Dominican monk of the thirteenth century. He was a great thinker whose genius covered so many fields that he came to be known as 'the Universal Doctor.' In his *'Boke of Secrets of Albartus Magnus of the Vertues of Herbs, Stones and certaine Beastes,*' he wrote about the use of the Periwinkle as a love potion ingredient.

> *'Perwynke when it is beate unto pouder with*
> *worms of ye earth wrapped about it and with an*
> *herb called houslyke, it induceth love between*
> *man and wyfe if it bee used in their meales'*

Stomach-turning though mashed earthworms might sound, all sorts of ingredients have been used since the days of the Ancients in order to work the magic of Venus. Human discharges and the reproductive parts of animals have been especially popular in charms and potions right up until fairly recent years. As you will see, the dividing line between Folk Medicine and Folk Magic was just about at its most blurred in the area of fertility, potency and attraction.

Mothers' Milk or human breast milk was highly sought after as a vehicle for the preparation of love potions. The Romans considered the milk from a mother who had just borne a male child to be the most effective.

Blood expressed from the Placenta, or afterbirth, was used by the Ancient Egyptians as an ointment when mixed with pomegranate juice. The belief was that it could impart a beauty to the skin which none could resist.

Menstrual Blood was regarded as 'bad' or 'evil' in many cultures. As a result, menstruating women were often barred from certain activities or places, lest they cause bewitchment in a similar way to the effect of the Evil Eye. Crops and medicinal plants were thought to be particularly vulnerable.

To the Romans, however, the uterus came to be regarded with veneration. The logic was that since it was the site of conception, development and birth, it had to be directly connected with the very life essense itself. Blood, one of the four vital fluids, which flowed periodically from a healthy woman was therefore thought to be a highly precious and potent fluid. Indeed, it was even believed that lightning and thunderstorms could be quelled merely by a menstruating woman baring her body during the storm.

An ointment made from menstrual blood from a woman who had borne children was considered to provide a certain cure for male impotency when rubbed on a male's genitals. It was also believed to produce powerful erections and enhance a man's love-making skills.

Seminal Fluid has also been regarded as a potent love-charm in cultures as distant in time and space as Ancient Greece and nineteenth century Scotland. A mixture of honey and seminal fluid made into a cake was regarded as a sure way of ensuring devotion.

IMPORTANT NOTE – THESE ANCIENT IDEAS ABOUT LOVE POTIONS MADE FROM HUMAN FLUIDS ARE MENTIONED FOR INTEREST, BECAUSE THEY WERE ACTUALLY USED IN FOLK PRACTICE. IN THE MODERN WORLD WITH THE THREAT OF HIV AND AIDS, THEY SHOULD NOT EVEN BE CONSIDERED.

Animal organs As mentioned above, it is a sad fact that innumerable animals have been sacrificed since the days of Antiquity, in order to make fertility and love potions. Hyaenas were highly regarded by the Romans, since it was believed that the animal was capable of changing its sex every year.

A hyaena captured during the full moon, especially if it was in the sign of Gemini (and the Moon spends approximately two and a quarter days in each Zodiacal constellation) was thought to have immense venal powers. Its genitals eaten in honey were considered a wonderful aphrodisiac.

The female hyaena fared no better with the Romans. Powdered hyaena uterus combined with sweet pomegranate freshly taken in wine was thought to prevent all gynaecological problems. It was also thought to make a woman supreme at love-making.

According to Pliny, the Romans also considered a rooster or cock to have venal powers which were worth preserving as a Talisman. A champion fighting cock was used if possible. It was ritually slaughtered and its testicles removed. These were then wrapped in a small ram's skin pouch which was worn about the waist.

In rural parts of Scotland last century it was thought that an ointment made from the bile of a goat, being a fertile and potent creature, would enhance a man's virility if rubbed over the penis regularly.

An old Gypsy aphrodisiac, apparently of Hungarian origin, consisted of the powdered testicle of a horse taken in beer or wine.

Unicorn Horn has been a traditional ingredient in aphrodisiacs for many centuries. Of course, there is no such creature, so unfortunate species which possess a horn have been needlessly slaughtered in their millions. Sadly, there are still some parts of the world where trade in rhinoceros horns is still legal, so the slaughter continues!

Conception charms

The questions surrounding conception have hardly changed over the centuries. People want to know what they must do to be fertile. What they must do to prevent pregnancy. And what they must do to have a child of a particular sex. Nowadays people visit their physician or gynaecologist and have the armamenterium of high-tech Medicine to help them. In the past it was the wise woman of the village or a local Folk Medicine practitioner of some sort who may have been consulted.

History and statistics show that most ancient contraceptive techniques were ineffective, dangerous or hazardous to health. In my studies of Folk Medicine I have found little which has any chance of bettering the methods currently available in orthodox practice (and in this context I include methods which are regarded as Natural Fertility techniques of conception and contraception).

Gender selection, however is interesting because of the number of quaint and curious things that couples have done in order to try to preselect the sex of their child. A common belief, even to this day, is that if a child is conceived when the parents made love in one position, then the opposite sex could be conceived by adopting reversed positions.

In Yorkshire it used to be believed that if a couple wished for a male child, the man should wear a hat during intercourse. If a female was desired, then he should wear an apron. Note that the determination of gender was believed to rest with the male.

It was commonly believed in the times of the Greeks – and also is still believed by some folk in Britain today – that the right testicle produces sperm which create male children, while the left creates females. Accordingly, bandaging one testicle was thought to allow the other testicle to work better, thereby producing a child of the desired sex.

Whatever method was chosen, there would be a fifty per cent chance of success!

Pregnancy testing

Finally, I close this chapter with a Folk Medicine pregnancy test which was used by the Ancient Egyptians. A similar method, I am informed, was used in Yorkshire (with apparent success) in comparatively recent times.

When a woman suspects pregnancy she gets a small handful of wheat and a similar amount of barley and she mixes them in a bowl with equal quantities of dates and sand. In the morning, she squats over the bowl and passes her first urine of the day over the mixture (just enough to thoroughly moisten the mixture). She then puts it away under her bed for two days. When she looks at it after that time, if the seeds have sprouted then it indicates pregnancy. More than that, if only the wheat germinates, then it is said to indicate that the child is to be a boy. If the barley germinates, then a girl is to be expected.

Chapter Eight

Natural Tonics

'Diet cures more than the lancet.'
Don Quixote

Miguel de Cervantes

How well I remember the taste!

That spoonful of castor oil and malt that my brothers and I had to have every morning from the middle of Autumn. It was a common 'tonic' that many of the youngsters in our town had to endure in order to stave off the coughs and colds of the Scottish winter.

Tonics have been prepared by people since Medicine began. Essentially, they are remedies which are thought to 'tone up' the system. People take them in order to hasten recovery from an illness, to boost the immune system, or to just give that bit more energy. At one time they were among the commonest prescriptions filled out by doctors. Nowadays they are not used at all, since they are considered to be nothing more than placebos.

The placebo again!

Well, it is true, the vast majority of the tonics which used to be used were probably quite ineffective. I have made a study of their ingredients and have to agree that few of them would have had any active pharmacological effect. Indeed, they were designed with that in mind. They belong to the era of Medicine when doctors were deliberately using inactive compounds which they knew would do no harm. Often the ingredients were chosen for their colour, odour, taste, viscosity or ability to fizz. With the best of intentions, these inactive tonics were prescribed with another aphorism of Hippocrates in mind – *'do no harm.'* And while the patient took the Medicine, the doctor waited for *Vis Medicatrix Naturae,* the healing power of nature to work its magic.

Now while the prescription of an inactive agent to 'fool' the patient is not considered ethical, the attitude that it is best to give nothing is not necessarily correct. As a doctor one sees this so often. Patients are told that 'Nature will take its course,' or that recovery will follow if you 'just get plenty of fresh air and good food.'

Again, I have to admit that there is some truth in such comments. Nature does take its course and fresh air and good food often do help. But on the other hand, Nature can take the easiest course which may make life difficult for the individual. Very often Nature needs a hand to get back on the best course.

The most damaging comment that people often come away with is, 'there's nothing that can be done, you'll have to live with it.' This is just not true. There is always something that can be done, something that can be tried. As a homoeopath I believe implicitly in this. To tell people that nothing can be done is therapeutic nihilism, no less.

But in this book I have no intention of extolling the virtues of Homoeopathy, or any other system of treatment. This is a book about Folk Medicine and the remedies which have been or are still being used by people today. In this context there are many natural tonics which do make people feel better and which are not placebos, in the derogatory sense implied by Conventional Medicine.

Natural Tonics

I use the word Natural to describe these tonics, because I wish to distinguish them from artificial chemical containing elixirs. The tonics I am going to consider have all been used in Folk Medicine all over the world. Nature, the best doctor of all, has provided them.

(Most of the herbs are warming in character, so you might care to make reference back to Chapter 5.)

HONEY – I start with this food, because it ranks top of my personal list of tonics. Not only that, but its pedigree is as long as you can get. When Hippocrates died there is a legend that they placed a bee-hive on his tomb, because he had extolled the value of honey for many years. The honey which the bees produced from that hive was thought to be especially effective.

You will note that throughout this book I have stated that honey can be used to take the bitterness off many herbal infusions and tisanes. It is raw sugar which the body can easily handle.

While diabetics should avoid all sugars and have their diets guided by their doctors, for mostly everyone else honey is an excellent food. In the convalescent stages of illness, or after an operation I think that a spoonful of honey twice a day can work wonders.

It can also be taken as '*Hydromel*', which is basically a mixture of honey, water, and various spices. The choice of spice is up to the individual's taste, but I rather like cinnamon. Mead is of course a fermented variety of hydromel. A small glass a day is a good pick-me-up after a debilitating illness.

GARLIC – This herb was known to the Ancient Egyptians, Chinese, Greeks and Romans. Garlic cloves have apparently been found in Ancient Egyptian tombs, left there as tonics to restore the Ka of the departed in the afterlife.

It is known that Garlic is a natural antibiotic and of value in hypertension and circulatory problems. It is excellent for the digestive system and is a good tonic in convalescent states. It can be taken several ways. It can be cooked in food, chewed as the clove, or swallowed as garlic capsules.

GINSENG – This herb (*Panax ginseng*) is my third favourite tonic. The botanical name Panax is derived from the Greek Panakes, meaning 'all-healing' – (similar to our word panacea). This is a warming herb which really does lift one's energy. It is extremely bitter and may benefit from the addition of a spoonful of honey or some chopped liquorice root. A cup morning and evening is the recommended dosage.

CIDER VINEGAR – This remedy was made famous by Dr D.C.

Jarvis, in his book Folk Medicine, which was first published in the 1950s. Dr Jarvis practiced in Vermont for some fifty years, during which time he studied Folk Medicine. He concluded that two teaspoonfuls of Cider vinegar and two spoonfuls of honey in a glass of water at each meal works as a natural tonic. He particularly felt that it worked well in arthritic conditions.

I would certainly accept that this is an excellent tonic which is very useful in some arthritic sufferers. I would counsel care, however, if someone suffers from stomach trouble, since the vinegar being acidic, can cause dyspepsia or a flare-up of a peptic ulcer.

KELP – This tonic agent has a remarkable reputation. It is a seaweed (*Fucus vesiculosis*), which has been used as a laxative, a tonic, a slimming agent and a thyroid gland stabiliser. It is rich in Iodine.

I have found this to be an effective aid in rheumatic disorders and a good all round tonic. It is readily available in health shops in tablet form. It is not one for prolonged self treatment, however. It should be taken under the advice of a health professional.

Incidentally, it is another agent which was advocated by Dr D.C. Jarvis.

LINSEED OIL – This tonic is one which I have found to be very effective for easing the tiredness and flushing of the menopause. It is derived from Flax (*Linum usitatissimum*) and is rich in phyto-oestrogens. It is available in capsule form from most health shops, the dosage being one to three capsules a day. It is a remedy which was known to Culpeper.

ANISEED – (*Pimpinella anisum*) This is an excellent digestive tonic and appetite stimulant. The seeds can be taken in an infusion, or a glass of the liqueur once a day can be taken if preferred!

BASIL – (*Ocimum basilicum*) This is an excellent restorative when exhausted. A sprig of basil leaves infused in a pint of water.

CARROT JUICE (*Daucus carota*) Although these are not easy to juice, the effort is well worthwhile. A glass of this tonic juice as and when one needs a pick-me-up works well indeed.

CAYENNE – *(Capsicum minimum)* When a bit of extra zest or '*pep*' is needed, try adding a pinch of cayenne pepper to a herbal tisane.

RASPBERRY LEAF – *(Rubus idaeus)* The tonic effect of Raspberry leaf tea upon the female womb is well known in the last weeks of pregnancy.

Oh yes, but what about castor oil and malt? – you may well have asked. Well quite frankly, I still remember the taste and couldn't bring myself to extoll its virtues!

Chapter Nine

The Monk, The Blacksmith and The Farmer's Wife

Medicine is a science which hath been, as we have said, more professed than laboured, and yet more laboured than advanced; the labour having been, in my judgement, rather in circle than progression.

Sir Francis Bacon

Medical Circles

It is said that Hippocrates, the father of Greek Medicine, spent the latter part of his life teaching on the Island of Kos. Sitting under a plane tree (which is allegedly still there) surrounded by his students he delivered his wisdom in short aphorisms. A collection of these, simply entitled *the Aphorisms*, formed one of the main texts of Medicine for almost two millennia. The very first aphorism began, 'Life is short, the Art (of Medicine) is long...'

By this Hippocrates meant that it takes a lifetime for a man to learn Medicine, but even then it will have advanced and will keep advancing after he has gone. Medicine should continue to evolve with greater and greater discoveries resulting in better health, less suffering and longer life. At least, that is what Hippocrates predicted would happen.

It may be, however, that Sir Francis Bacon was nearer the truth when he cynically remarked that Medicine moves in circles rather than in a straight onward line of progress.

As we have seen throughout this book Medicine does seem to move through phases of magic, religion and science. This is because society moves through these phases itself. Yet the phases are not independent entities. Simply because we live in a scientific age does not mean that people no longer believe in religion or magic. Far from it. We all have our own beliefs. For some people these beliefs may be in accord with the current day teachings. For others the belief may be based upon what they feel is right for them. This may be the logical, rational, scientific view and attitude which is fostered and thrust upon us by Western developed society. The attitude which compartmentalises our lives and tends to reject that which cannot be explained by science as mere superstition. Alternatively, it could be the innate, basic human belief in magic and religion. And of course, there are shades of belief between these two extremes.

The point is that society is made up of individuals. Every human group is made up of people who will agree and disagree at times. In Medicine we see this ebbing and flowing phenomenon all the time. In the twenty years that I have been involved in clinical practice I have seen treatments come and go. As a student I was taught some things and told that unless I alluded to them in examinations, I would risk failure. As I write now, some of those theories have been rejected completely. When I was a young medical house officer in hospital I used standard drugs and treatments, only to find that twenty years down the line they are considered too dangerous to use. I have seen new 'wonder-drugs' come along, work extremely well for a while, then develop horrendous side-effects.

This is the effect of fashion in Medicine. True, the fashions change when research studies prove efficacy or inefficacy. But it is also true to say that counter-trials by different researchers often fail to confirm the research findings of the first workers. In this respect the science of Medicine does often work in circles in that treatments come, then go, then come back again.

At the deeper more important level, it is unquestionably true that the developed world has by and large freed itself from plagues and the major infectious diseases. Vaccines and drugs have gone a long way towards achieving this, but the contribution of improved water supplies, sewage disposal and simple hygiene have been vital. The scenario that now seems to be played out in Western Medicine today is one of damage limitation. Although we have reduced the infectious diseases, we have replaced them with the degenerative conditions of arteriosclerosis, arthritis and auto-immune diseases. Technology now allows us to maintain people in comatose states for years and to replace fluids, organs and an increasing number of joints.

Many people have become disillusioned by this approach and have re-examined their attitude to health care. As a result there has been an increasing interest in Natural and Complementary Medicine over the last two decades. This has seen a flourishing of many seemingly new therapies and a mushrooming of Natural and Complementary Medicine Colleges and professional bodies. Public opinion alone has forced the medical profession to climb down from a very anti-Complementary Medicine stance and accept that it does have a place in todays health marketplace.

Folk Medicine to Natural Medicine

When one looks at the individual Natural or Complementary Therapies one thing stands out. They can all trace their origin to some past wisdom or aspect of what was once established medical practice. Although that method may not have been practised by the orthodox profession for many years, centuries in some cases, in virtually every case there will have been people who have kept it alive. In other words, the therapies have been rediscovered from the great pool of Folk Medicine practice.

Let us look at some examples.

Aromatherapy – oils have been used by the Ancient Chinese and Egyptians, the Arabs, Greeks and Romans. Country people have been using various oils for generations, yet the method is attributed to Rene Gatefosse, during the First World War. Undoubtedly he systematised it, yet it has been practised in various forms across the world almost continuously since the days of the Ancients.

Auriculotherapy – this therapy involves stimulating points upon the ear, usually with needles in a manner similar to that of

Acupuncture. It was developed in the 1950s by Dr Paul Nogier, a French doctor, after he observed that many of his patients had strange cauterisation marks on their ears. They had in fact been treated by a local Folk practitioner for sciatica, with good result. In his researches Nogier discovered that the method had been practised by sailors for centuries and that there was evidence that some methods were used by the Ancient Egyptians.

Chiropractic and Osteopathy – these are two methods of manipulative medicine which have both been derived from the age-old tradition of bone-setting. Every culture since the Stone Age has had its bone-setters.

Herbal Medicine – as we have seen in earlier chapters, herbs have supplied man with medicine since the dawns of time. Whether people have lived in highlands, planes, rainforests or jungles, plant sources have been available to them. No-one can doubt either the value of herbal medicine or the benefit which has been gained from the extraction of drugs from herbs.

We saw in Chapter Five how Western Herbal Medicine has developed from the circuitous root it took when emigrants from all over Europe settled across the American frontier to amalgamate their traditional practice with that of American Indian herbal medicine.

Homoeopathy – the basic principle of Homoeopathy is *similia similibus curentur* – let like be cured by like. Although Hippocrates is always said to have acknowledged that one could either treat by similars or by opposites, it is Dr Samuel Hahnemann (1755–1843) who is recognised as the originator of Homoeopathy. The word comes from the Greek *homoios*, meaning 'like', and *pathos*, meaning '*suffering*'.

In treating a patient a Homoeopath matches up the symptoms of the patient to the symptom-profile of a substance which would produce the same pattern of symptoms when given to a well person. The appropriate substance, be it of animal, mineral or vegetable origin, is given in a very reduced and potentised form, to stimulate the body to fight the disease.

One cannot but help notice the similarity of the basic principle to that of Sympathetic Magic remedies which have been used in Folk Medicine over the centuries. Although Hahnemann is said to have arrived at the concept in a logical manner through rational experimentation, it is highly likely that he was aware of Folk practices involving this sympathetic principle.

Naturopathy – the method of Medicine which is based upon 'nature cure,' dates back to Hippocrates. Another of his aphorisms was, 'For everything in excess is opposed to Nature.'

Essentially, he believed that when people abuse their systems they risk illness. He also taught that physicians did not cure disease, but that they assisted Nature. The truth of this is absolute. Unless the individual has sufficient vitality then no medicine on Earth will bring about a cure.

The Nature Cure movement is said to have begun in the mid-nineteenth century, originally under the direction of Vincenz Priessnitz, the 'father of Hydrotherapy,' who set up a clinic in Germany. Johannes Schroth followed suit in Austria, as did prominent physicians like Henry Lindlahr in the USA.

Many of the Naturopathic principles are so basic and commonsensical that one suspects them to be almost innate. Bathing a muscle or joint that is strained, avoiding food when nauseated, resting after exertion, these are all naturopathic principles. They are also things which the elders of the families have been advising for years, just as they were themselves advised.

Reflexology – another '20th Century' Complementary Therapy has been attributed to the work of Dr William Fitzgerald in the years before the First World War. In fact, foot massage for treating various body problems has been practised by the Ancient Egyptians, Chinese and Indians.

Radiesthesia and radionics – these Complementary methods of Medicine are methods of absent healing. They derive from dowsing over a blood spot, urine sample or specimen of saliva. They illustrate yet another principle of magic belief – that once some fluid (or hair sample, etc) has been part of the body, it will continue to operate a psychic link with the individual. It is the basis of many types of magic belief, such as the malevolent use of wax dolls in Voodoo.

The Monk, the Blacksmith and the Farmer's Wife

In the British Isles during the Medieval Age people really had three potential levels of care. They could treat themselves or be treated by the local wise person. They could go to a barber, surgeon or grocer-spicer. Finally, they could visit a monastery and receive treatment from the monks.

The spread of Christianity had gradually absorbed the beliefs about sacred places and wells, as we have seen, through the expediency of blessing them. As the monasteries grew up they became natural centres of healing, because the Church effectively 'controlled' the places previously associated with healing. Not only that, but since the monasteries maintained libraries and provided rudimentary teaching, it was inevitable that within their walls they would became the custodians of the literary texts of Medicine. These texts would include the traditional herbals and leech books containing the accumulated knowledge from Celtic, Saxon and Teutonic sources, as well as translated texts of Greek medical wisdom which had been kept alive by absorbtion into the Arab world. Many of these latter works were brought back by returning Crusaders.

The Reformation and the Dissolution of the Monasteries by King Henry Vlll effectively removed this source of medical care. A medical profession had begun to be established with the Barber-Surgeons and the Apothecaries providing a form of general practice for the middle classes, while the university trained physicians offered the nobility an elite service. The poor and those living in rural areas were presented with problems. More than ever before they would have had to depend upon self-help and the knowledge of local wise people.

With the Dissolution of the Monasteries, vast numbers of monks would have found themselves destitute, or forced into life as mendicants. Some with skills in healing would undoubtedly have used their expertise as they travelled about the countryside. And inevitably, some of their lore would drift into the pool of oral tradition that is Folk Medicine.

Some monks would have developed expertise in bone-setting, others in herbal medicine. Still others would have other callings which they would be able to put to good use. Among these would be skills as farriers and blacksmiths.

It seems curious to us nowadays to think that at one time people went to barbers to have minor surgery performed on them. Even more curious, however, is the medical ability which black-smiths seemed to have. But then again, blacksmiths almost inevitably became the experts on dealing with the ailments of animals. That being the case, it was but a short step towards the treatment of human beings.

Iron symbolises strength, of course, so that when people wanted to become strong they would look for a means of absorbing the strength of the metal. The blacksmith's *bosh,* the cooling trough for quenching all sorts of red hot iron, was considered to teem with strength. Accordingly, drinking a tonic made from bosh water was considered useful for anaemia, convalescent conditions and all debilitating illnesses.

A third generation blacksmith was thought to have special powers of healing. Because of their strength and knowledge of horses joints, many were much sought after as bone-setters.

Not only that, but because much of his material became magnetic, it was thought that it would hold special curative powers. Magnetised nails were considered wonderful amulets to protect one against the Evil Eye and against rheumatism and the ague.

Of course, not everyone could travel to the blacksmiths. In really rural communities some person would tend to accumulate medical lore. Most cultures tell the same story – that person was usually a woman. A woman associated with the land, with experience of having children and of delivering other women's children. She would have knowledge of herbs and somehow draw on the rich oral tradition of Folk Medicine as it was passed onto her from her parents, just as they had learned from theirs. And so in time she too would teach her knowledge to her offspring. And they would some-times pass on their lore to others, perpetuating the flow from that great pool of Folk Medicine.

And that – is where I came in!

SECTION TWO

The Remedies
Appendix 1 The Saints
Appendix 2 The Herbs

The Remedies

'Would you have a settled head,
You must early go to bed:
I tell you, and I tell't again,
You must be in bed at ten.'

Nicholas Culpeper

As I stated in the introduction, it has not been my intention to produce either a text-book of Folk Medicine or yet another Family Herbal. This is a written record of remedies which have been or are still being used in different parts of the world by people as a first line of self help. Many of the remedies date back to Antiquity when magic was an integral part of Medicine. Others are relatively new and have merely filtered into the common pool of Folk Medicine from the advancing tide of orthodox practice. Common to the majority, however, is the fact that they have been kept alive mainly through word of mouth.

In the first section of the book we looked at guiding principles in the selection of remedies. In this section, I have compiled an A–Z of common conditions, symptoms and problems for which there are known Folk Medicine remedies. In order to simplify matters I have also divided the remedies into five basic types:–

1) Invocations to different Saints.
2) Magico-Medicine remedies. These are often extremely old treatments, based upon magical beliefs.

3) Doctrine of Signatures. These are also very old, some dating back at least a thousand years, to the days when a plant, animal or mineral's appearance, smell or taste gave it a special 'signature.'

4) Traditional remedies. Here we find all manner of remedies from all epochs.

5) Waters. Here we look at the use of healing waters, spas and bath treatments.

While the book is primarily intended to interest the reader, there may be some who would care to try out the remedies themselves. To them I must emphasise a few points:–

• This book is not intended to replace medical advice.

• I have endeavoured to describe only herbal remedies which are generally considered safe. There are many more used in Folk Medicine which I have deliberately excluded from this work, because I feel they are too toxic to risk inclusion.

• No dosages are given. This is quite deliberate, since this is not a text-book of Medicine or Herbalism. The remedies are taken from Folk Medicine practice which has always been an inexact and an oral art. To impose artificial dosages would have been quite inappropriate with the spirit of the subject. Having said that, in the matter of herbal treatments a good rule of thumb is to use about an ounce of the herbal matter to three-quarters of a pint to make a strong infusion; an ounce to a pint to make a refreshing tisane. When using woody barks or roots then a decoction is made, rather than an infusion. The difference is that the herb is simmered in the solution for a certain time, usually fifteen minutes.

• We have an ecological duty to our fellow creatures and to endangered plant species. Many of the Magico-Medicine remedies are barbaric and are mentioned only for interest. Similarly, many herbs are (or should be) protected by law. I would therefore advise individuals to use only herbs that they can grow in their own herb garden, or which they can obtain from health shops or reputable herbal suppliers. This of course also ensures that the correct herb is chosen!

• PREGNANT WOMEN SHOULD TAKE AS LITTLE AS POSSIBLE – AND BE GUIDED BY THEIR OWN HEALTH ADVISER.

Abscess, boils and pimples

INVOCATIONS – St Blaise, St Anthony, St Benedict.
MAGICO-MEDICINE – The talismanic charms of St Benedict and St Anthony were considered to be protective against such infections. The charm and incantation of Abracadabra set the trend for all Magico-Medical spells.

> *Thou shalt on paper write the spell divine*
> *ABRACADABRA called in many a line,*
> *Each under each in even order place,*
> *But the last letter in each line efface,*
> *As by degrees the elements grow few,*
> *Still take away but fix the residue,*
> *Till at the last one letter stands alone,*
> *And the whole dwindles to a tapering cone.*
> *Tie this about the neck with flaxen string,*
> *Mighty the good 'twill to the patient bring,*
> *Its mighty potency shall guard his head*
> *And drive disease and death from his bed"*

Among precious gems, the garnet was thought to be highly effective in ridding the body of boils and absesses. Diamonds and Pearls are also said to increase the body's defences against infections of all sorts.

Up until the last war it was customary in most parts of Great Britain to bake bread or Hot Cross buns on Good Friday. Some of that bread was kept for the rest of the year, in case anyone fell ill in the household. If they did – with a infection – then some of the breadcrumbs were given as an infusion. If there was a skin infection like an abscess, then a poultice using some of that bread might be used. A similar custom was used at Christmas times.

DOCTRINE OF SIGNATURES – A tisane or infusion of poplar or aspen bark (shiver trees) drunk twice a day when feverish was recommended.

TRADITIONAL REMEDIES – Garlic is a natural antibiotic which has been used since Antiquity. Garlic cloves can be crushed and applied directly to the infected part. They can also be placed in a sock, which actually allows absorption through the skin. This method can actually work almost as well as taking cloves of garlic by mouth.

Hawthorn (Crataegus monogynova) – a poultice made out of the leaves is good for drawing boils and splinters which have been slow to form or come out.

Oats (Avena sativa) – a poultice is excellent for drawing infections. I have used this for treating the severe discomfort of mastitis in the post natal period.

A paste of soap and sugar will often draw all sorts of minor skin infections.

Urine poultices used to be advocated by many folk healers. Linen soaked with warm, freshly passed urine was laid over the inflamed part, reputedly with good effect.

Honey applied directly to abscesses is a treatment used throughout the world. It was used by the Ancient Egyptians and was advocated by Hippocrates.

Another traditional remedy is *Romany Balm*. This has been used for centuries by European Gypsies for all sorts of boils and minor cuts and grazes. It is made from 3 ounces of pig fat (especially from around the kidneys), one ounce of horse-hoof clippings, a houseleak and one ounce of grated Elder bark. The ingredients were simmered for half an hour together, then strained into a container. When cooled this provided a useful stock of ointment.

Finally, Sphagnum Moss (Sphagnum cymbifolium) has been a favourite remedy from American Frontier Medicine, where it was used by the American Indians. Gypsies also advocated its use, especially when it was soaked in the juice of a herbal antiseptic such as garlic or onion.

WATERS – Bathing in thermal waters or muriated waters was considered a good way of dealing with infections of the skin. Simply having salt baths or soaking the part in salt water may soothe many superficial skin infections.

IMPORTANT NOTE Although many Folk remedies may work well for such infections, there is always a potential danger of infection spreading to affect the whole system. This condition of septicaemia is dangerous, so a medical opinion should not be unduly delayed. A course of antibiotics may be necessary.

Accidents

INVOCATION – St Benedict and St Christopher.
MAGICO-MEDICINE – The talismanic charm of St Benedict was considered a protection against accidents. This was later supplanted by the St Christopher medallion, which is today one of the commonest charms in Folklore.

The caul achieved universal fame as a protection against drowning. Sailors and fishermen would be prepared to spend considerable amounts to buy one to protect them while, at sea. It was also believed that the man who carried one would never suffer from sea-sickness or scurvy.

Wearing ivory is thought to protect the wearer from sudden injury and accidents.

Aching legs

MAGICO-MEDICINE – A piece of cork in the bed is said to ease aching legs which prevent sleep at night.
TRADITITIONAL REMEDIES – Cayenne pepper (Capsicum annum), a warming remedy is useful for aching legs. About a quarter of a teaspoon is taken in a cup of water twice a day for as long as felt necessary.

A sage bath is also an excellent restorative for aching muscles and joints. This can be combined with heating a handful of salt then sprinkling it over a dry flannel. Wrap the flannel about the legs and leave on for about ten to fifteen minutes. It can be repeated if necessary.

WATERS – A Mustard bath is an old and favoured remedy for aching feet and legs.
(PLEASE SEE CHAPTER 6 REGARDING MUSTARD BATHS).

Acidity

INVOCATIONS – St Timothy of Lystra, the protector of those with weak stomachs.

TRADITIONAL REMEDIES – It is obvious to anyone troubled by stomach acidity that they are worse whenever they lie flat. Propping the head end of the bed up on books to raise it two or three inches may make all the difference.

Drinking milk generally gives immediate relief, although it is generally very short-lived.

Eating a raw potato, as one would an apple is an excellent remedy for excess acidity. I cannot recommend this method too highly.

Infusions of Dandelion, Gentian, Meadowseet and Yellow Dock are all traditional remedies for easing excess acidity. I would particularly commend Meadowsweet.

Grated Oak bark (Quercus robur), half an ounce in a pint of boiling water, makes a drink that looks like whisky or brandy. A small glassful daily after food is useful for easing heartburn and stomach acidity. It is traditionally known as *Decoctum Quercus*.

WATERS – *Simple Alkaline Waters, or simple soda waters*, are waters mainly containing sodium bicarbonate. Because of the alkalinity of the waters these were understandably considered beneficial in countering the effects of excess acidity in the body. They were, therefore, recommended for stomach ulcers and dyspepsia, and for bladder troubles and urinary stones.

Acne

MAGICO-MEDICINE – Transference magic was often invoked against this condition, since people thought that the characteristic lesions were caused by minute worms which had 'black heads'. It was thought that they blocked the skin pores. One Magico-medical remedy involved squeezing a few of the 'blackheads' and forcing them into the mouth of an animal, or allowing a dog to lick them away.

TRADITIONAL REMEDIES – A useful poultice was made from Oats (Avena sativa) soaked overnight in cream. To this mixture the juice of a lemon was squeezed. This was then applied as a face pack which was left to harden. It was then washed off in warm water and the skin dabbed dry.

In the Highlands of Scotland 'the Black Heids' were removed by squeezing them out with the key of a pocket watch. The skin was then cleaned with a mixture of whisky and carbolic soap.

Drinking one's own urine every morning for nine days was often advocated, as was using some of the urine to wash in every night.

WATERS – *Indifferent Waters or simple thermal springs,* are the waters which contain relatively little in the way of minerals, so that they are almost pure water. Usually they arise from warm springs and are naturally carbonated. Generally, such spas were places that people went to bathe as well as to take the waters internally. The effect of the escaping gas was thought to stimulate the skin. Often these spas were found in hilly regions. They were thought to be especially good for chronic skin disorders.

Addiction – (to alcohol and tobacco).

INVOCATIONS – St Amand, the patron saint of brewers and inn-keepers.

MAGICO-MEDICINE – A particularly noxious remedy for alcoholics was to drink beer or wine in which a frog had been drowned. (Frogs are amphibians, so they do need air).

Wearing a bloodstone is said to help one accumulate enough will power to deal with an addiction!

TRADITIONAL REMEDIES – Mainly these play a part in easing the anxiety and craving as one withdraws from the habit. Chamomile (Anthemis nobilis), is an excellent relaxant and sedative. An infusion of the flowers makes a bitter herbal tea which is made palatable with spearmint, honey or grated liquorice root.

Gentian (Gentiana lutea), is a well known bitter, useful for anxiety states, such as can occur on withdrawal from alcohol or tobacco. Stock can be made by infusing an ounce of the grated root in a pint of boiling water. Two tablespoonfuls three times a day is the usual dosage when needed.

Chewing the stem of the Greater Plantain (Plantago Major) when the craving for a smoke is upon one may reduce the craving.

Tobacco substitutes have also been advocated to help the individual withdraw from the tobacco. There are several different ones which can be smoked in a pipe or taken in cigarette form. They usually contain Coltsfoot, Buckbean, Euphrasia, Betony, Rosemary, Thyme and Lavender.

WATERS – *Sulphinated Waters, or bitter waters,* are waters containing Epsom or Glauber's salts (respectively hydrated forms of magnesium and sodium sulphate). Because of this chemical composition they produce a sulphur smell, a bitter taste and an aperient effect. Taken internally, these were thought to be especially good for all liver problems, including those caused by a dependence on alcohol.

Anaemia

INVOCATIONS – St Alban and St John the Baptist.

MAGICO-MEDICINE – Wearing amethysts, bloodstones or rubies are thought to be useful for anaemia and blood disorders.

TRADITIONAL REMEDIES – an ounce of Burdock root, boiled in a pint of water for five minutes then allowed to cool made a stock solution of a traditional blood tonic. A tablespoonful twice a day was reckoned to enrich and strengthen the blood.

Blacksmiths were thought to have cures for blood disorders, by virtue of the iron with which they worked. Water drunk from the the trough in which horseshoes and tongs had been quenched was thought to enrich the blood.

Carrots are traditionally given for anaemia. They are grated and taken as a large side-portion with a meal every day.

Nettle tea, four times a day is said to stimulate blood cell production. Yarrow tea is said to have a similar action when two cups are taken daily.

WATERS – Spa treatments were often recommended at resorts known for their Chalybeate waters, or iron waters. Inevitably, these were all thought to be tonifying for anaemia and other disorders of the blood.

Anger

MAGICO-MEDICINE – wearing a sardonyx next to the skin is said to balance the hot-headed temperament.

TRADITIONAL REMEDIES – Chamomille (Anthemis nobilis), is an excellent relaxant and sedative. An infusion of the flowers makes a bitter herbal tea which is made palatable with spearmint, honey or grated liquorice root.

Angina

INVOCATIONS – St Valentine and St Teresa of Avila.

TRADITIONAL REMEDIES – An old Yorkshire remedy designed to prevent the Angina producing effect of cold winds, was to sprinkle brown sugar into hot bacon fat (from the bottom of the frying pan) and cover a sheet of brown paper with it. When it was cool it was applied to the chest and left under the vest. The cold winds were thought to be unable to penetrate this.

Anus – see Haemorrhoids

Anxiety

INVOCATIONS – St Bartholomew and St Dympna, the patron saint of the insane and those who suffered with nervous problems.

MAGICO-MEDICINE – Wearing amethysts and sapphires is thought to alleviate general anxiety. Agates are also said to be good for those with little self-confidence.

DOCTRINE OF SIGNATURES – a cup of an infusion of the bark of Aspen or Poplar trees once a day. These were 'shiver trees' thought useful when one trembled like a leaf with anxiety.

TRADITIONAL REMEDIES – Chamomile (Anthemis nobilis), is an excellent relaxant and sedative. An infusion of the flowers makes a bitter herbal tea which is made palatable with spearmint, honey or grated liquorice root.

Gentian (Gentiana lutea), is a well known bitter, useful for anxiety states. Stock can be made by infusing an ounce of the grated root in a pint of boiling water. Two tablespoonfuls three times a day is the usual dosage when needed.

Hawthorn (Crataegus monogynova), a warming herb, also called *Hagthorn*, is useful for fearful conditions when taken as a tisane twice a day. A heaped spoon of the hawthorn flowers and leaves is used to make a pot of the tisane.

WATERS – *Indifferent Waters or simple thermal springs*, are the waters which contain relatively little in the way of minerals, so that they are almost pure water. They were thought to be especially good for nervous and excitable conditions of the nervous system.

Appetite

TRADITIONAL REMEDIES – Hawthorn (Crataegus monogynova), a warming herb, also called *Hagthorn*, is useful for stimulating the appetite when taken as a tisane twice a day. A heaped spoon of the hawthorn flowers and leaves is used to make a pot of the tisane.

Horse-radish (Cochlearia armoracia), a warming herb, is used as a remedy to stimulate the appetite. One or two roots, grated down and taken daily in several divided doses before meals. Taking bread at the same time will reduce the heat in one's mouth.

Yarrow (Acillea millefolium), also called *Bloodwort, Woundwort and Staunch-weed*, a warming herb, is excellent for stimulating the appetite when taken as a herbal tea.

WATERS – *Simple Alkaline Waters, or simple soda waters*, are waters mainly containing sodium bicarbonate. They were recommended for stomach ulcers, dyspepsia and poor appetite.

Arthritis

MAGICO-MEDICINE – There was an old highland belief that the metal from a decomposed coffin worn as a medallion would cure and prevent gout and rheumatism. Wearing a ruby is thought to be helpful for those suffering from arthritis and rheumatism.

DOCTRINE OF SIGNATURES – A tablespoonful of an infusion of St John's Wort three times a day is useful for the acute pain of a flare-up of arthritis.

TRADITIONAL REMEDIES – The Romans used to use Urtication, the practice of thrashing the affected part with nettles in order to raise nettle-rash wheals. It produces a counter-irritation to the pain and does give short-lived relief.

Another remedy which dates back to their time is the practice of burying ones painful joint in the ground, near to an ant-hill. The resultant bites from the ants produce an even more intense inflammatory counter-irritation which is said to be extremely effective. Please do note, however, that this method could be extremely dangerous if the individual is allergic, so it is mentioned purely out of historical interest.

A very common remedy advocated by Gypsies and country folk in Yorkshire was to mix cow dung in vinegar and boil the mixture. A thick poultice was then wrapped around the swollen part, the poultice being replaced every day or two. It was said to work equally well on horses, cattle and humans.

A related remedy was to mix cow dung in the individual's own urine and boil the mixture. A thick poultice was applied as above.

In some parts of Scotland and the North of England, arthritis sufferers used to be advised to use warm urine soaks around their painful joints and to drink a cup of urine night and morning.

Cayenne pepper (Capsicum annum), a warming remedy, is used for arthritis. About a quarter of a teaspoon is taken in a cup of water twice a day for as long as felt necessary.

Fennel (Foeniculum vulgara), a warming herb, is useful for helping rheumatism. The leaves can be chewed.

Feverfew (Chrysanthemum parthenium), also called Nosebleed, is useful for arthritis. The flowers made into an infusion and taken as a herbal tea are beneficial twice a day. Also, if the leaves are made into a poultice then they are said to be useful for relieving painful, swollen joints.

Nettle (Urtica urens), the Common Stinging Nettle, a warming herb, also called Bad Man's Plaything, and Sting-leaf, as a herbal tea is also well known as a useful treatment for arthritis and rheumatism.

Cider Vinegar and honey. This remedy was made famous by Dr D.C. Jarvis, in his book Folk Medicine, which was first published in the 1950s. Dr Jarvis practiced in Vermont for some fifty years, during which time he studied Folk Medicine. He concluded that two teaspoonfuls of Cider vinegar and two spoonfuls of honey in a glass of water at each meal works well in arthritic conditions. (NOTE – this should not be tried if there is a history of stomach trouble).

A compress or poultice of boiled Bladderwrack (Fucus vesiculosus), or Kelp is excellent for painful gout or acutely inflamed arthritic joints.

WATERS – For someone particularly troubled by arthritis of the hips, a Sitz-bath three or four times a week is to be recommended. It will often work particularly well if a handful of dried nettle leaves are added to the hot part of the bath.
(PLEASE SEE CHAPTER 6 REGARDING SITZ-BATHS).

Asthma

MAGICO-MEDICINE – The skins of long-chested animals, such as *hares*, were thought to be capable of transfering the lung-efficiency of the animal to an asthma sufferer. The skin was simply placed over the sufferer's chest while they slept.

Wearing an opal next to the skin is said to soothe the spasms of the lungs.

TRADITIONAL REMEDIES – Elecampane (Inula helenium), also called Wild Sunflower and Horseheal, is useful for respiratory catarrh and for clearing up bronchitis when taken as a herbal tea. One teaspoon of the ground or shredded root is soaked overnight in a pint of water. A tablespoon or a small wineglass three times a day is taken to help ease the problem.

Backache

TRADITIONAL REMEDIES – hanging by ones arms from a

door for as long as one can, is a very old and effective form of self-traction.

A bath to which Elecampane, the whole herb, has been added is extremely good and helps many people.

Cider Vinegar and honey may work well (see ARTHRITIS).

Opodeldoc. You may remember that I told you about a patient of mine who was given 'Deldoc' by an old farmer friend of his. He had used this remedy just as it had been passed down to him. Note that this remedy was originally used by Paracelsus, so it is of considerable antiquity (even if the ingredients I now cite are the modern counterparts!) It was made from half a pint of vinegar, half a pint of Turpentine, half a pint of methylated spirits, the white of two eggs and quarter of a pint of liquid soap.

The ingredients were mixed thoroughly, bottled and left to stand for two days. The liniment was then ready for use and could be applied to the back every four to six hours when necessary.

IMPORTANT NOTE All skin applications can be irritant to people with sensitive skins. No-one with a skin irritation should contemplate using this.

Bad Breath – see Halitosis

Baldness – see Hair loss

Bed-wetting

INVOCATIONS – St Dympna, the patron saint of the insane and those who suffered with nervous problems.

MAGICO-MEDICINE – An amulet fashioned from the dried bladder of a mouse was thought to be effective when worn about the neck.

TRADITIONAL REMEDIES – The Ancient Egyptians believed that this could be cured by eating roast mouse or mouse pie.

The Romans used urtication, thrashing the insides of the legs with nettles. This was more punitive than therapeutic, I imagine.

An ingenious mediaeval alarm consisted of tying a frog or a toad between the legs of the individual when they went to bed. If they started to pass water, the frog would awaken, start croaking and waken the individual and the household!

A table spoonful of honey after the evening meal will often bring about a dramatic change.

Black eye

DOCTRINE OF SIGNATURES – Green Oil of Charity (Adder's Tongue) applied to the bruise night and morning. Also Calamint or Bruisewort, whose juice was like bile or the colour of resolving bruises. Its leaves were soaked in wine then applied to the bruised area. Lesser Celandine was also used as a poultice made from the whole herb.

Another traditional remedy was based upon the Doctrine of Signatures. This was the use of raw meat to be placed over the black eye. A beaf steak is the meat most usually cited.

Blisters

TRADITIONAL REMEDIES – Soaked cabbage leaves placed over the blistered area will soothe the discomfort and act as a good buffer against further trauma. They should be replaced every few hours.

Greater Plantain leaves placed over a blistered area will soothe the blisters. They can also be used preventively by putting them inside one's socks prior to walks.

Blood disorders

INVOCATIONS – St Alban.

MAGICO-MEDICINE -Wearing amethysts, bloodstones or rubies are thought to be useful for anaemia and blood disorders.

DOCTRINE OF SIGNATURES – St John's Wort (Hypericum perforatum), also called Holy Herb, Balm to the Warrior's Wound, Touch and Heal. This herb in mediaeval times was thought to have been imbued with healing powers because St John the Baptist had reputedly worn a girdle of the plant while he was in the wilderness. Its red flowers and curiously perforated leaves were thought to represent the blood of the saint and its ability to cure wounds. An infusion of the finely chopped flowers, drunk in a tablespoon three times a day, was used to cure all types of minor haemorrhage, and to treat all types of blood disorder.

TRADITIONAL REMEDIES – An ounce of Burdock root, boiled in a pint of water for five minutes then allowed to cool made a stock solution of a traditional blood tonic. A tablespoonful twice a day was reckoned to enrich and strengthen the blood.

Blacksmiths were thought to have cures for blood disorders, by virtue of the iron with which they worked. Water drunk from the the trough in which horseshoes and tongs had been quenched was thought to enrich the blood.

WATERS – Spa treatments were often recommended at resorts known for their Chalybeate waters, or iron waters. Inevitably, these were all thought to be tonifying for anaemia and other disorders of the blood.

Bone disorders

MAGICO-MEDICINE – Wearing a ruby next to the skin was thought to help bone problems.

WATERS – Spa treatments were often recommended for bone disorders which were far more common in the last century when nutrition was less adequate and when people did not expose their bodies to sunlight. Calcareous Waters, or lime waters were understandably thought to be valuable in bone deficiency conditions, like rickets, osteomalacia and osteoporosis (although the latter was not precisely diagnosed as such in those days).

Breast problems

INVOCATIONS – St Agatha.

TRADITIONAL REMEDIES – Celery tisane is often helpful for painful breasts around the period. A cup twice a day.

According to American Frontier Medicine, Mastitis could be treated by scraping carrots and softening them on a fire shovel, or the hot plate of a stove. If they were then applied to the inflamed part they eased the pain and helped to reduce the inflammation.

This was regarded as a good remedy for many inflammatory problems (see EYE PROBLEMS, SINUSITIS).

IMPORTANT NOTE – It is vital that dangerous breast conditions are not missed, so a medical opinion should be sought.

Bronchitis

MAGICO-MEDICINE – Opal worn next to the skin is said to help all lung conditions.

An old Irish Folk remedy consited of taking the wool from a black sheep and laying it out like a small mat. Onions were then fried in oil or fat and laid over the wool. When it had cooled enough, it was applied to the sufferer's chest.

DOCTRINE OF SIGNATURES – Lungwort or Oak Lungs, a teaspoon of the dried herb in a cup of water three times a day may ease the symptoms.

Garlic (Allium sativum) was thought to be good for all conditions affecting 'tubes' since it has a hollow stem.

TRADITIONAL REMEDIES – Goose Grease rubbed over the chest was a common old Yorkshire remedy for bronchitis sufferers.

Elecampane (Inula helenium), also called Wild Sunflower and Horseheal, is useful for respiratory catarrh and for clearing up bronchitis when taken as a herbal tea. Mustard (Sinapsis alba), a warming herb, also called Gold Dust, can clear catarrh and bronchitis when a weak infusion is sipped sparingly throughout the day. Too much, however, and it will overheat the stomach and induce nausea.

Thyme added to a hot water inhalation bowl will often soothe the cough.

Bruises

DOCTRINE OF SIGNATURES – Green Oil of Charity (Adder's Tongue) applied to the bruise night and morning. Also Calamint or Bruisewort, whose juice was like bile or the colour of resolving bruises. Its leaves were soaked in wine then applied to the bruised area. Lesser Celandine was also used as a poultice made from the whole herb.

TRADITIONAL REMEDIES – Opodeldoc used to be advised, provided there was no breakage of the skin. See BACKACHE.

Witch Hazel (Hamamelis virginiana), as 'extract of witch hazel' applied directly to sphagnum moss and applied to a bruise is an excellent bruise-soother.

Comfrey (Symphytum officinale), also called Knitbone, has been used since Antiquity. It was a standard preparation in the days of the monasteries. Applied as an ointment it is superb for easing all bruises and sprains.

Arnica (Arnica montana), known in homoeopathy as 'the Healer' is world famous as a remedy to apply to all bruises and sprains.

Burns

MAGICO-MEDICINE – burns, scalds and abrasions could apparently be dealt with by the following incantation:–

> 'There came two angels from the north.
> One was fire and one was frost.
> Out, fire! In frost!
> In the name of the Father, Son and Holy Ghost.'

DOCTRINE OF SIGNATURES – The Common Stinging Nettle, the whole herb made into a lotion or an infusion is useful for easing the pain of superficial burns and scalds.
TRADITIONAL REMEDY – Apparently, the Crusaders used to use Sweet Chestnut (Castanea vesca) leaves which were soaked in hot water to soften them, then allowed to cool. They were then placed across the burned surface. This will soothe the burning sensation.

Cabbage (Brasica) leaves similarly soaked are also beneficial.

Catarrh

DOCTRINE OF SIGNATURES – Lungwort or Oak Lungs, was thought to be useful for all sorts of respiratory problem, especially those associated with increased catarrh. A teaspoon of the dried herb in a cup of water three times a day is recommended.

TRADITIONAL REMEDIES – Betony (Stachys Betonica), also called Bishopswort, Wood Betony and Sentinel of the Woods, a few leaves infused as a tea, drunk twice a day is considered useful for catarrhal headaches, sinusitis and muzzy-headedness. Elecampane (Inula helenium), also called Wild Sunflower and Horseheal, is useful for respiratory catarrh and for clearing up bronchitis when taken as a herbal tea. Garlic (Allium sativum), is a long-established treatment fro catarrhal problems. Hyssop (Hyssopus officinalis), is used as an expectorant for troublesome respiratory catarrh. An infusion of the flowers as a herbal tea twice or three times a day is recommended until symptoms settle.

Honey and Liquorice Elixir is an old fisherman's remedy (see under COUGH).

WATERS – a Sitz bath two or three times a week may help, especially if a handful of Elecampane leaves are added to the hot part of the bath
(PLEASE SEE CHAPTER 6 for SITZ BATHS).

Chapped hands

DOCTRINE OF SIGNATURES – Oil of St John's Wort, prepared from simmering the chopped flowers in oil, is useful for all sorts of painful chaps and cuts and sores on the hands and fingers.
TRADITIONAL REMEDIES – In many country areas it was believed that chapped hands could be quickly cured by passing one's urine over them night and morning.

Goose Grease, the fat from the goose, is almost thought of as a specific cure for chapped hands in rural parts of Yorkshire.

Romany Balm (see ABSESSES AND BOILS above) was advocated by Gypsies.

Chilblains

DOCTRINE OF SIGNATURES – Green Oil of Charity (Adder's Tongue) applied to the chilblain night and morning.
TRADITIONAL REMEDIES – *Romany Foot Ointment* also has an ancient pedigree. It was made from 3 ounces of animal fat (traditionally pig fat), one ounce of Flowers of Sulphur, one ounce

of Olive Oil. These were simmered gently for half an hour and well mixed, then poured into a container. It was considered excellent for treating and preventing chilblains, corns and all sorts of foot problems.

A slightly more modern remedy was advocated by the celebrated Mrs Beeton

'Bake a common white turnip and scratch out the pulp, mix it with a tablespoon of salad oil, one of mustard and one of grated horse-radish. In this way form a poultice and apply it to the chilblains on a piece of linen rag.'

Walking barefoot in the fresh snow whenever feasible is said to be a specific for chilblains. No more than a few seconds should be done on the first day or two, gradually increasing to a minute or two.

As a preventive, the individual might try running in the dew covered grass in the Summer and Autumn.

Childbirth

INVOCATIONS – St Margaret of Antioch and St Erasmus were invoked to aid the birth itself. St Brigid was invoked on behalf of the newborn infant.

MAGICO-MEDICINE – Before modern midwifery and obstetrics started to reduce infant and maternal mortality rates, Magico-medical remedies were frequently resorted to. This is understandable since pregnancy and childbirth were very much in the lap of the gods.

Amulets and talismans against the Evil Eye, witches and malign influences have been used for many centuries across the globe. An old Italian and Sicilian one consisted of a fragment of the umbilical cord from a previous healthy child.

Pregnant women were considered to be particularly vulnerable to all sorts of evil and malign influences, visible or invisible. For this reason, in several cultures a pregnant woman is well nigh kept in seclusion for the whole of her pregnancy.

The delivery place was generally specially prepared by having all of the doors open and any knots in ropes, strings, threads or hair untied. This, it was believed, would ensure the free passage of the baby and prevent the umbilical cord from getting knotted around the child's head.

Upon being born the baby was inspected for birth marks which could indicate that some malign influence had touched the child while it was in the womb. The kiss of a virgin was said to remove any such evil, as did the precaution of rubbing the birthmark with saliva.

Haemorrhage in the newborn baby and a postpartum haemorrhage in the mother in the first fortnight were very common in the past. To counter the first, it was common practice in Scotland to tie the umbilical cord with red thread. To counter the latter problem for the mother, a red flannel, towel or cloth was hung over the end of the labour bed.

In some African tribes it is traditional to place a small heap of cow dung near to the mother in labour. The belief is that the child will smell how healthy its father is, thereby ensuring a swift delivery.

Wearing a sapphire is said to prevent bleeding problems after the birth of a baby.

TRADITIONAL REMEDIES – Gypsies advise taking wild raspberries in the last week of pregnancy and at the start of labour to ease any pain. In addition, Raspberry leaves (Rubus idaeus) taken as a tisane in the last week or so of pregnancy is said to strengthen the tone of the womb.

IMPORTANT NOTE – There are other herbal remedies which have been used in Folk Medicine, but Raspberries are the only ones which I feel are safe for use without individual guidance from a health professional.

Circulatory problems

MAGICO-MEDICINE – Wearing a ruby is said to improve the circulation.

DOCTRINE OF SIGNATURES – Garlic (Allium sativum) was thought to be good for all conditions affecting 'tubes' since it has a hollow stem.

TRADITIONAL REMEDIES – Cayenne pepper (Capsicum annum),

a warming herb, is used for sluggish circulation. About a quarter of a teaspoon is taken in a cup of water twice a day for as long as felt necessary.

Garlic (Allium sativum), also known as Gypsy's Onions, is good for the circulatory system and blood pressure. A whole clove chewed daily, or proprietory garlic pills can be taken. Parsley is worth chewing afterwards in order to counter the characteristic pungent garlic odour (see above, DOCTRINE OF SIGNATURES).

Hawthorn (Crataegus monogynova), a warming hertb, also called Hagthorn, is generally considered tonic to the heart and circulatory system. The leaf buds when chewed taste like Pepper and Salt, yet another country name.

Cold

DOCTRINE OF SIGNATURES – Catmint or Catwort, is eaten by cats when suffering from infections. It promotes sweating, so was considered useful for colds.

TRADITIONAL REMEDIES – Hyssop (Hyssopus officinalis), a warming herb, is used as an expectorant and as a diaphoretic, a preparation which induces sweating during an infection. An infusion of the flowers as a herbal tea twice or three times a day is recommended.

Sage (Salvia officinalis), taken like hyssop is a powerful diaphoretic (a remedy that promotes sweating). Gargling with an infusion of the leaves eases a sore throat and hastens the passage of catarrh.

Onions have been considered helpful for many generations. A peeled and cut onion was thought to be useful for preventing the spread of colds when someone in a household is infected. One was simply left on a mantelshelf in each of the rooms. Another remedy said to nip a cold in the bud, consists of peeling an onion and making several cuts through it. Then quickly dip it into a jug of boiled water for about five seconds. The liquid should then be strained and kept. The entire jugful of this water should then be sipped throughout the whole day. Hopefully, the cold will not have developed by the next day.

To prevent an infection from a cold or from the effect of cold winds, an old Yorkshire remedy was to sprinkle brown sugar into hot bacon fat (from the bottom of the frying pan) and smear it over a sheet of brown paper.. When it was cool it was applied to the chest and left under the vest.

WATERS – a Mustard foot bath every other day during the cold may ease the symptoms.

Cold sores

MAGICO-MEDICINE – Transference magic played a great part in many remedies for these painful lesions. Snails or slugs were used in one Magico-Medicine remedy, wherein a snail or slug was rubbed over the lesion then sealed in a bottle which was buried in the garden. As the creature died, so did the cold sore fade away.

TRADITIONAL REMEDIES – Marsh Cudweed (Gnaphalium uliginosum) is a well known herb which when made into an infusion, makes an excellent remedy for dabbing on cold sores.

Colic

INVOCATIONS – St Erasmus.

MAGICO-MEDICINE – According to Sicilian Folk Medicine when a child was born, the sensible parents asked the midwife to give them a small segment of the umbilical cord. This was carefully wrapped in cloth and put away for safety as a cure for colic. It could either be used as an amulet which was rubbed over the abdomen, or pulverised and taken internally in wine.

A ruby worn next to the skin is said to protect against colic.

DOCTRINE OF SIGNATURES – Ginger tea or chewing a little of the raw root before meals seems to ease colic.

TRADITIONAL REMEDIES – Chamomile (Anthemis nobilis), a cooling herb can ease the spasms of irritable bowel syndrome and colic. An infusion of the flowers makes a bitter herbal tea which is made palatable with spearmint, honey or grated liquorice root.

Self-Heal (Prunella vulgaris), also called All Heal, Sicklewort and Hookweed. An infusion of its flowers, drunk by the tablespoon three times a day seems to ease irritable bowel cramps.

WATERS – For someone particularly troubled by colic pains from the Irritable Bowel Syndrome, a Sitz-bath twice a week is to be recommended. It will often work particularly well if a handful of chamomille flowers and leaves are added to the hot part of the bath. (PLEASE SEE CHAPTER 6 REGARDING SITZ-BATHS).

Complexion

DOCTRINE OF SIGNATURES – Walnut oil or lotion is considered useful for the skin.

TRADITIONAL REMEDIES – The Ancient Egyptians used pomegranate in several cosmetics. The juice of the fruit is said to be very beneficial to the skin.

Elder (Sambucus nigra), also known as Boon Tree, is said to help the complexion generally. An infusion of the Elder flowers, one ounce per pint of water, makes *Elderflower Water* which makes a good skin wash which stimulates the skin. This used to be known as *Aqua Sambuci*.

An old English rhyme contains a belief in the virtue of Hawthorn dew as a complexion enhancer:

> *That fair maid*
> *Who, at break of day,*
> *Goes to the fields*
> *On the first of May,*
> *And washes in dew*
> *From the hawthorn tree*
> *Shall ever afterwards*
> *Beautiful be.*

Dandelion tea taken regularly is an old remedy which is said to enhance the complexion.

An old Highland face pack is made from two handfuls of oatmeal, soaked for three hours, plus a teaspoon of freshly squeezed lemon juice and just enough cream from the top of milk to make a pack. Cucumbers placed over the eyes are excellent for soothing tired eyes. They are thought to prevent wrinkling. Fresh tea bags are also advocated as a natural skin toner, when placed over the eyes.

Conjunctivitis

MAGICO-MEDICINE – An emerald worn next to the skin is said to protect against eye problems.

DOCTRINE OF SIGNATURES – Eyebright or Clear-Eye, makes an excellent eye lotion. The whole herb is boiled in three-quarters of a pint of water. The cool lotion may be used three or four times a day to bathe the eyes.

TRADITIONAL REMEDIES – Fresh garden dew bottled and rubbed over the eyelids two or three times a day is an old Scottish remedy for easing sticky and painful eyes.

IMPORTANT NOTE – An acutely red and painful eye might be caused by iritis or glaucoma. Both of these need an urgent medical opinion.

Constipation

DOCTRINE OF SIGNATURES – Couch Grass or Dog Grass is eaten instinctively by dogs and is found to open the bowels. The bruised roots were boiled in wine, a glass of which taken in the evening and at bedtime should open the bowels.

Liquorice root, either chewed directly or taken as an infusion with honey is a gentle worker of the bowel.

TRADITIONAL REMEDIES – Cinnamon (Cinnamonum zeylanicum), a warming herb, is useful for constipation. A quarter teaspoonful in water twice a day, for as long as felt necessary.

Fennel (Foeniculum vulgara), a warming herb, is useful for settling constipation. The leaves can be chewed.

Dandelion (Taraxicum officinale), also called Devil's Milk-pail, is a well known bitter which has been used as a laxative for centuries. The leaves can be freely chewed, although over-indulgence can cause nausea. An infusion of the leaves taken as a herbal tea is also quite a useful way of taking the herb. As yet another alternative, the dried roots, ground and powdered can make a coffee substitute.

WATERS – Sulphinated Waters, or bitter water spas specialised in this problem. Taken internally they cleansed the bowel.

A Sitz-bath twice a week, containing a herb such as fennel,

dandelion or chamomille in the hot part, will often stimulate a sluggish bowel.

IMPORTANT NOTE – Any sudden alteration in bowel habit could be caused by a serious bowel condition for which a medical opinion and diagnosis is necessary. An opinion should not be delayed by injudicious self-treatment.

Corns

INVOCATIONS – St Christopher, the patron saint of travellers.

TRADITIONAL REMEDIES – a Sage footbath quickly eases the footsore walker, especially if afflicted with corns.

Romany Foot Ointment was considered excellent for treating and preventing corns and for all sorts of foot problems (see CHILBLAINS).

WATERS – A Mustard bath is an old and favoured remedy for corns.

(PLEASE SEE CHAPTER 6 REGARDING MUSTARD BATHS).

Cough

MAGICO-MEDICINE – Spiders were thought to be useful in getting rid of coughs. An old remedy was to place a live spider in a matchbox and wear it around the neck. As the spider died, so was the cough supposed to disappear.

A similar example of Transference Magic was used in Scotland where live frogs were placed in a bag and tied inside the chimney. As they croaked away and died, so would they take away a cough in the house. This was a classic magical cure for whooping cough.

TRADITIONAL REMEDIES – Honey and Liquorice Elixir is an old fisherman's remedy. Quarter of a pint of white vinegar, a couple of tablespoonfuls of running honey, quarter of an ounce of good black liquorice and one lemon. The finely cut liquorice is added to the vinegar which is heated slowly. The honey and lemon are added when the mixture is boiling. It is then allowed to cool. A teaspoonful when the cough is troublesome may be taken. This is said to be good for both dry coughs and congested coughs. It is also very good for catarrh.

Another old country cough syrup was easily made by slicing half a dozen onions and placing them in a sieve above a bowl. They should then be sprinkled with a liberal quantity of brown sugar. The juice which runs off is collected and can be taken a spoonful when necessary to soothe an irritant cough.

Coltsfoot (Tussilago farfara), also known as Coughwort is perhaps one of the best known traditional cough mixtures. A handful of the flowers should be infused in a pint of water and left to cool. A glass or cupful, sweetened with liquorice root or melted honey three times a day will often soothe an irritant cough.

Cramps

INVOCATIONS – St Pancras.

MAGICO-MEDICINE – Pliny, writing in AD 77 tells us that that a rabbit or hare's foot could cure cramp.

Coffin handles, nails and hinges were all thought to alleviate cramp pains anywhere in the body when made into a ring.

In many parts of England and Scotland people used to (and still do) carry cramp bones. These could be the patella or knuckle-bone of a sheep, or hare. Worn as an amulet they could protect from the cramp pains of rheumatism and gout. Placed under the pillow they were believed to cure all sorts of muscular pains overnight.

In Yorkshire, the wearing of an eel-skin garter was (and still is) advocated in rural areas to prevent and cure cramp and rheumatism. It was hoped that the suppleness of the eel would transfer itself to the afflicted joint and cramped muscles. Another ubiquitous remedy throughout country areas of England was to place a piece of cork under the blankets to prevent cramp throughout the night.

A ruby worn next to the skin is said to protect against cramps.

With recent interest in pyramids and pyramidology, many people place a small pyramid under their bed and claim relief from cramp.

TRADITIONAL REMEDIES – Chamomile (Anthemis nobilis), a cooling herb which is good at removing and preventing the pain of nocturnal cramps. An infusion of the flowers makes a bitter herbal tea which is made palatable with spearmint, honey or grated liquorice root.

WATERS – For someone particularly troubled by night cramps, a Sitz-bath twice a week is to be recommended. It will often work particularly well if a handful of chamomille flowers and leaves are added to the hot part of the bath.
(PLEASE SEE CHAPTER 6 REGARDING SITZ-BATHS).

Cuts and grazes

INVOCATIONS – St Giles.
DOCTRINE OF SIGNATURES – Oil of St John's Wort, prepared from simmering the chopped flowers in oil, is useful for all sorts of painful chaps and cuts and sores on the hands and fingers.
TRADITIONAL REMEDIES – a compress made from spiders webs was used by the Ancient Romans and the American Indians. Similarly, Sphagnum Moss (Sphagnum cymbifolium) has been a favourite remedy from American Frontier Medicine, where it was used by the American Indians for infections and cuts and grazes. Gypsies also advocated its use, especially when it was soaked in the juice of a herbal antiseptic such as garlic or onion.

Romany Balm (see ABSESSES AND BOILS above) was advocated by Gypsies.

Comfrey (Symphytum officinale), also called Knitbone and Pigweed, makes an excellent healing ointment for cuts and grazes. A handful of the dried leaves should be pound in a pestle and mortar and mixed with vegetable fat or cold cream. It can be applied several times a day.

Cystitis

MAGICO-MEDICINE – A bloodstone worn next to the skin is said to protect against bladder and kidney problems.
DOCTRINE OF SIGNATURES – Burdock root soaked in water overnight to make an infusion, was used for all urinary problems. A cup or glass was taken twice a day.
TRADITIONAL REMEDIES – Parsley Piert (Alchemilla arvensis), also called Breakstone or Colicwort, taken as an infusion of the whole plant twice a day is useful for soothing the discomfort associated with many bladder and urinary problems.

Parsley (Petroselinum crispum), taken as a daily tisane made from the dried or fresh leaves is a well-established urinary soother and diuretic.

Couch Grass or Dog Grass has been found useful in cystitis and as a laxative. The bruised roots were boiled in wine, a glass of which was taken in the evening and at bedtime. Care has to be taken in case too much is taken – remembering its laxative action!

Barley water (Hordeum pratense) is a remedy which is still commonly advised by Family Doctors. A handful of pearl barley is scalded in a pint of water and simmered for twenty minutes. It is then strained and flavoured with lemon juice. A tumblerful three times a day will usually ease the discomfort of cystitis.

WATERS – For someone troubled by recurrent episodes of cystitis (provided that the diagnosis has been confirmed), then a Sitz-bath twice a week is to be recommended. It will often work particularly well if a handful of chamomille flowers and leaves, or lavendar herbs are added to the hot part of the bath.

(PLEASE SEE CHAPTER 6 REGARDING SITZ-BATHS).

Deafness

MAGICO-MEDICINE – Wearing an article of jewellery made of Onyx is said to improve the hearing.

TRADITIONAL REMEDIES – Instilling warm urine into the ears was advocated in many country areas in order to improve the hearing.

IMPORTANT NOTE – Wax may not be the only cause of hearing problems. A health professional should be consulted.

Depression

INVOCATIONS – St Dympna, the patron saint of the insane and those who suffered with nervous problems.

MAGICO-MEDICINE – wearing a carnelian is thought to be useful in lifting a depression. Amber, garnets and jasper are also thought to ease depression when worn as jewellery, preferably next to the skin.

Drinking from a silver vessel was thought to ease or prevent depression.

TRADITIONAL REMEDIES – Chamomile (Anthemis nobilis), is an excellent relaxant and sedative which can lift the mood. An infusion of the flowers makes a bitter herbal tea which is made palatable with spearmint, honey or grated liquorice root.

Gentian (Gentiana lutea), is a well known bitter, useful for anxiety states and mild depression. Stock can be made by infusing an ounce of the grated root in a pint of boiling water. Two table-spoonfuls three times a day is the usual dosage when needed.

IMPORTANT NOTE – Depression can be a serious condition which can worsen spontaneously. A professional opinion should be sought early.

Diarrhoea

DOCTRINE OF SIGNATURES – Ginger tea or an infusion of the grated root taken several times a day is said to rapidly stop diarrhoea.

IMPORTANT NOTE – Any sudden alteration in bowel habit could be caused by a serious bowel condition for which a medical opinion and diagnosis is necessary. An opinion should not be delayed by injudicious self-treatment.

Dizziness

MAGICO-MEDICINE – Drinking wine to which a few drops of a black cat's blood had been added (cats having excellent balance) was thought to cure troublesome dizziness.

TRADITIONAL REMEDIES – Eating kelp soup was advocated in coastal areas. This may have had a Doctrine of Signatures association, since kelp comes from the sea which can, of course, cause sea-sickness and dizziness. Having said that, taking a course of kelp under the supervision of a professional might be worth trying.

Dreams – (see Medical divination, Chapter 3)

Earache

INVOCATIONS – St Cornelius.
MAGICO-MEDICINE – Removing some wax from a painful ear, a sufferer was advised to rub it on a piece of bread and throw it outside for the birds. The pain was thought to be transfered away as the bird flew off with the bread.

Eczema

DOCTRINE OF SIGNATURES – Castor Oil Plant or Christ's Hand, was thought to have a direct healing effect on the skin when the oil was placed over the affected area. Walnut oil or lotion is also useful for very dry, flaking eczema.
TRADITIONAL REMEDIES – Figwort (Scrophularia nodosa), also called the Scrophula Plant, Brownwort, Carpenter's Herb and Poor Man's Salve, is used as an ointment for eczema. The whole herb or leaves boiled in water or oil, made a useful mode of treatment. Alternatively, the soaked leaves can be used as a poultice.
   Romany Balm (see Absesses and boils above) was advocated by Gypsies.
WATERS – *Indifferent Waters or simple thermal springs,* are the waters which contain relatively little in the way of minerals, so that they are almost pure water. Usually they arise from warm springs and are naturally carbonated. Generally, such spas were places that people went to bathe as well as to take the waters internally. The effect of the escaping gas was thought to stimulate the skin. Often these spas were found in hilly regions. They were thought to be especially good for chronic skin disorders.

Epilepsy

INVOCATIONS – St Antony, St Cornelius, St Dympna, St Valentine, St Vitus.
MAGICO-MEDICINE – This condition was very common at one time, possibly because so many communities were closed, with consequent genetic inbreeding. Many magico-medical remedies were employed throughout the world. An example of Transference

magic involved taking hair and nail clippings and wrapping them in a small bag with a coin. These were then taken and buried at a point where three lands met (ie a cross-roads), ideally at midnight. If anyone happened to come across the bundle, then they would have the illness transferred to them.

Another magico-medical treatment involved drinking from a healing vessel fashioned from a skull. Pliny, writing in AD 77 gives an early instance of this method. Some sources say that the skull had to be that of an ancestor, others that it had to be that of a murdered innocent. If the water was from a holy well, then the magic worked better. If the well was little known about, then the magic worked best of all.

A commonly held belief in many lands was that a hangman's noose could cure all manner of problems above the neck. Accordingly, if one wore a string made up from a few strands from a hangman's noose, then fits could be controlled.

In addition, an old highland belief was that the metal from a decomposed coffin worn as a medallion would cure epilepsy.

Wearing Lapis Lazuli has been advocated since the days of the Ancient Egyptians, who called it the Stone of Heaven. It was thought to be good for preventing eye problems and epilepsy.

Finally, wearing the T-shaped cross of St Antony as an amulet was thought to be protective against having fits.

Erysipelas

INVOCATIONS – St Antony, St Benedict, St John.
MAGICO-MEDICINE – This painful condition was understandably associated with many amulets, talismans and spells. The amulets of St Antony and St Benedict were considered valuable protectives against both Erysipelas and Shingles.

Black cats, being associated in the popular mind with magic were considered to hold a cure for Erysipelas. The ear of a black cat was cut off and the blood allowed to drip over the painful part. Then, using some of the blood as ink, the patient's name was written on paper or parchment, then thrown into the fire.

Fortunately, Donkeys had a less sacrificial role to play, due to their being regarded as 'holy animals'. The black cross on their backs, reputedly due to having carried Jesus, was thought to be a natural source of healing. Some hair clippings were taken boiled in water and painted over the affected area.

MEDICAL NOTE – Erysipelas is an acute feverish condition associated with an area of painful, spreading erythema or redness. It is due to a bacterial infection. In past days it could spread rapidly and cause spticaemia. It was very probably confused with other medical conditions like shingles.

Eye problems

INVOCATIONS – St Thomas, St Dunstan.

MAGICO-MEDICINE – Black cats, because they could see in the dark, were often used grotesquely for the treatment of failing vision. The head of a pure black cat was burned to ashes. Once a day a small quantity of the ashes were rubbed between the fingers and then rubbed in the eyes. This Magico-Medical remedy seems to have been used quite freely around the countryside in the sixteenth and seventeenth centuries.

In the highland moors of Scotland, where adders were common, so-called *Adder stones* were eagerly sought after. These were thought to have been produced by the concretion of adder spit. Small Adder stones were believed to be effective against eye problems.

Wearing Lapis Lazuli has been advocated since the days of the Ancient Egyptians, who called it the Stone of Heaven. It was thought to be good for preventing eye problems and epilepsy. Emerald and quartz are also said to be protective for the eyes.

DOCTRINE OF SIGNATURES – Eyebright or Clear-Eye makes an excellent eye lotion. The whole herb is boiled in three-quarters of a pint of water. When cool it may be used three or four times a day. It is said to improve and clear the vision.

TRADITIONAL REMEDIES – Fresh garden dew, bottled and rubbed over the eyelids two or three times a day is an old Scottish remedy which is said to be good for all sorts of eye inflammations.

According to American Frontier Medicine, many eye inflammations could be treated by scraping carrots and softening them on a fire shovel. If they were then applied over the closed eyes and over the cheekbones they eased the pain and helped to reduce the inflammation. This was regarded as a good way of soothing many inflammatory conditions. (see BREAST PROBLEMS, SINUSITIS).

Fainting

INVOCATIONS – St Antony, St Cornelius, St Dympna, St Valentine, St Vitus.

MAGICO-MEDICINE – A tendency to faint may well have been considered as a sort of epileptic tendency in the past, so the same remedies would have applied.

TRADITIONAL REMEDIES – To revive someone from a faint people used to have first recourse to a bottle of smelling salts. Virtually every household at one time kept a small bottle of Sal Volatile in the medicine cabinet. It produces an extremely pungent smell. Smouldering paper was also used if smelling salts were not to hand.

IMPORTANT NOTE – Above all else, a patient should not be raised from the lying position until they recover spontaneously. Trying to raise someone before they are physiologically ready could result in them actually having a convulsion, since the brain would be temporarily deprived of oxygen. This may account for many people in the past having been misdiagnosed as having epilepsy.

Alcohol after a faint is not a good idea, so do not give brandy!

Fears

INVOCATIONS – St Dympna, the patron saint of the insane and those who suffered with nervous problems.

MAGICO-MEDICINE – most amulets and talismans were made to protect, hence they were active against fear.

Wearing a charoite stone is thought to be almost a specific protection against panic and terror. A turquoise was said to be particularly helpful for those too frightened to talk in public. According to the old saying:

> *"If you wear a turquoise blue,*
> *Success will crown whate'er you do."*

Sympathetic magic was used by making some sort of preparation from the feared object and consuming it, in order to consume the fear. Thus, a fear of spiders could be overcome by eating ground spiders in a cake. Also, taking the properties of a fearless creature, eg the heart of an ox, or the blood of an ox was thought to give one protection from fear.

TRADITIONAL REMEDIES – Chamomile (Anthemis nobilis), is an excellent relaxant and sedative. An infusion of the flowers makes a bitter herbal tea which is made palatable with spearmint, honey or grated liquorice root.

Gentian (Gentiana lutea), is a well known bitter, useful for anxiety states. Stock can be made by infusing an ounce of the grated root in a pint of boiling water. Two tablespoonfuls three times a day is the usual dosage when needed.

Hawthorn (Crataegus monogynova), a warming herb, also called Hagthorn, is useful for fearful conditions when taken as a tisane twice a day. A heaped spoon of the hawthorn flowers and leaves is used to make a pot of the tisane.

WATERS – *Indifferent Waters or simple thermal springs,* are the waters which contain relatively little in the way of minerals, so that they are almost pure water. They were thought to be especially good for nervous and excitable conditions of the nervous system.

Feet ache

WATERS – A Mustard bath for twenty minutes is an old and favoured remedy for aching feet and legs.
(PLEASE SEE CHAPTER 6 REGARDING MUSTARD BATHS).

Feet burning

TRADITIONAL REMEDIES – A Sage footbath quickly eases the footsore walker.

Romany Foot Ointment was considered excellent for treating and preventing all sorts of foot problems (see CHILBLAINS).

Fever

INVOCATIONS – St Anthony, St Benedict, St Genevieve.

MAGICO-MEDICINE – Pliny, the Roman historian writing in 77 AD tells us that a green lizard should be enclosed in a small earthenware jar and worn as an amulet in order to dispell a fever.

In the Highlands of Scotland last century, a ritual mock burial was carried out with children suffering from a feverish condition. The child was taken into a churchyard and layed down on the grass. Pieces of turf were placed upon the body and the head, then removed. The process was repeated three times. The theory was that by burying the illness, but resurrecting the child, the illness would be left in the mock grave.

Applying the opened bodies of pigeons which had been cut open while they were still alive was a standard magico-medical remedy often used in Elizabethan and Jacobean times. Dr John Hall, the son-in-law of William Shakespeare, records that in 1632 he himself was debilitated by '*a moderate flux......and then a deadly burning fever.*' He took to bed and had the live pigeon treatment applied to himself in order to '*draw down the vapours.*'

Tying a piece of red thread around the throat when smitten with a feverish condition was at one time common throughout Great Britain. The thread had to be red.

DOCTRINE OF SIGNATURES – An infusion of the powdered bark of Aspen or Poplar trees was given twice a day.

Flatulence

MAGICO-MEDICINE – Wearing an opal next to the skin was thought to help all manner of digestive problems.

TRADITIONAL REMEDIES – Peppermint,

WATERS – *Simple Alkaline Waters, or simple soda waters*, are waters mainly containing sodium bicarbonate. Because of the alkalinity of the waters these were understandably considered beneficial in countering the effects of excess acidity in the body, which often causes flatulence.

Freckles

TRADITIONAL REMEDIES – Elder (Sambucus nigra), also known as Boon Tree, is said to help the complexion generally. An infusion of the Elder flowers, one ounce per pint of water, makes Elderflower water which makes a good skin wash which stimulates the skin. This used to be known as *Aqua Sambuci*.

Rubbing freckles with lemon juice is said to lighten freckles through a slight bleaching action.

IMPORTANT NOTE – any freckle or mole which seems to undergo a change in size, deepening of pigment, or which starts to grow hairs or bleed, MUST be checked by a doctor.

Gall-bladder problems

MAGICO-MEDICINE – Wearing jasper is thought to prevent biliousness and gall bladder problems. Those at risk, traditionally women who are fair, fertile, well-proportioned and over the age of forty, are said to benefit from this stone.

DOCTRINE OF SIGNATURES – Burdock root soaked in water overnight to make an infusion. A glass or cup twice a day was thought to help gall stones, just as it did urinary gravel.

TRADITIONAL REMEDIES – Parsley Piert (Alchemilla arvensis), also called Breakstone or Colicwort, taken as an infusion of the whole plant twice a day is useful for soothing the discomfort associated with many gall bladder problems.

WATERS *Sulphinated Waters, or bitter waters,* are waters containing Epsom or Glauber's salts (respectively hydrated forms of magnesium and sodium sulphate). Taken internally, these were thought to be especially good for gall-stones and gall bladder problems.

Glands

MAGICO-MEDICINE – Swellings in the neck were referred to as Wens. They were usually either caused by a thyroid goitre or by glands in the neck from many causes. They were often treated by Transference Magic. One such remedy involved stroking the throat with a live snake nine times, then burying the snake alive in a bottle. As it died and decomposed, so it was thought that the wen would go away.

The Roman historian Pliny reports that glandular trouble would be cured if the hand of a corpse was placed on the troubled part. To be most effective, it was thought that the corpse had to be that of someone who had died prematurely.

A hangman's noose was also said to be effective in past times for curing swollen glands. It or some strands from the rope, were to be drawn across the goitre or wen nine times.

Goitre

MAGICO-MEDICINE – Swellings in the neck from enlarged thyroid glands were called Wens. These were extremely common in areas far removed from the sea. In England they were so common in the Peak District of Derbyshire that 'Derbyshire Neck' became a common description for the condition.

Wearing Topaz or Sapphire was thought to be helpful for helping goitres to reduce.

It was also commonly believed that the hand of a corpse could cure a wen. Accordingly, people with goitres would attend a wake in order to have the corpse's hand placed upon their neck.

Another common practice in rural areas was to take nine hairs from the tail of a stallion and make them into a plait. This was to be worn about the neck. When they eventually wore out, so the wen would resolve.

TRADITIONAL REMEDIES – Bladderwrack (Fucus vesiculosus), also called Kelp or Popper Sea-Weed tablets are said to have a beneficial effect upon the thyroid gland. Stimulating an underactive gland and sedating it when it is overactive. It is not one for self treatment, however. It should be taken under the advice of a health professional.

Gout

INVOCATIONS – St Andrew and St Gregory.

MAGICO-MEDICINE – It was an old highland belief that the metal from a decomposed coffin worn as a medallion would cure and prevent gout and rheumatism.

TRADITIONAL REMEDIES – Celery and Nettle tisanes taken twice a day may be helpful in easing the discomfort of gout.

Comfrey leaves soaked overnight and wrapped around the swollen joint is said to ease the discomfort of acute gout.

A compress or poultice of boiled Bladderwrack (Fucus vesiculosus), or Kelp is excellent for painful gout or acutely inflamed arthritic joints.

WATERS – Muriated Saline Waters, or simple salt water spas were thought to be beneficial. Bathing in them was thought to stimulate the skin, thereby having a beneficial effect upon disorders of the kidneys and conditions thought to be resultant from defective kidney function, such as gout.

Gravel

MAGICO-MEDICINE – A bloodstone worn next to the skin was said to protect against gravel.

DOCTRINE OF SIGNATURES – Burdock root soaked in water overnight to make an infusion. This was thought excellent to free one from urinary gravel, when a tablespoon was taken twice a day.

TRADITIONAL REMEDIES – Parsley Piert (Alchemilla arvensis), also called Breakstone or Colicwort, taken as an infusion of the whole plant twice a day is useful for soothing the discomfort associated with many bladder and urinary problems.

Parsley (Petroselinum crispum), taken as in infusion also has a long history of usage for urinary gravel. It was used by the monks of Annaghadown.

Gravel-Root (Eupatorium purpueum), also called Joe Pye Weed, is another traditional remedy for these symptoms. It was used a lot by American Indians and was a favoured herb in Western Frontier Medicine. An ounce of the whole herb in a pint of water should be infused. A wineglassful four or five times a day is said to be very effective.

WATERS – Muriated Saline Waters, or simple salt water spas were thought to be beneficial. Bathing in them was thought to stimulate the skin, thereby having a beneficial effect upon disorders of the kidneys, including urinary gravel.

Gum problems

MAGICO-MEDICINE – in country areas it was recommended that the painful gum should be scratched with a nail or jagged piece of wood found in a graveyard. The nail should then be hammered into a tree or the wood buried in an old grave. The gum problem would be transferred from the sufferer.

Agates have always been considered good for curing gum problems and easing infant teething.

TRADITIONAL REMEDIES – Oil of cloves is a good remedy for soothing the pain of a dental abscess or 'gum-boil.' A few drops are rubbed directly on the painful site.

In Scotland a small toddy is made up from a teaspoon of whisky and a half teaspoon of bown sugar and a couple of teaspoons of boiled water. A cotton wool ball is soaked in the toddy and applied to the painful area. This is not a remedy which should be given to children, of course!

Haemorrhoids

INVOCATIONS – St Fiacre.

DOCTRINE OF SIGNATURES – Lesser Celandine or Pilewort poultice made from the whole herb was applied to the haemorrhoids twice a day. Also Figwort or Carpenter's Herb (Poor Man's Salve) used in exactly the same way as Lesser Celandine.

TRADITIONAL REMEDIES – Witch hazel extract applied to sphagnum moss placed over the haemorrhoids is a remedy which was used in American Frontier Medicine.

WATERS – Sulphinated Waters, or bitter waters taken internally were thought to be especially good for all sluggish bowel problems and piles.

Hair loss

MAGICO-MEDICINE – an old Gypsy remedy consisted of making

an ointment from the fat of a hedgehog, two handfuls of Rosemary, two handfuls of nettle leaves and a few pinches of salt. This awesome mix was to be rubbed into the scalp twice a week.

The Romans favoured the organs of the ass with hair restorative powers. One remedy involved rubbing the shaven scalp with ashes from the burned genitals of the poor creature. Another remedy involved taking the ashes from a foal's generative organs and mixing them with one's own urine. The scalp was regularly annointed thus to produce a good head of thick hair which would not go grey.

TRADITIONAL REMEDIES – Rosemary and Nettle infusions used as a rinse when shampooing the hair are said to stimulate hair growth.

Halitosis

TRADITIONAL REMEDIES – Chewing parsley or a cinnamon stick sweetens the breath.

Hands

DOCTRINE OF SIGNATURES – The Greater Plantain or Englishman's Foot, was considered useful for disorders of the hands and feet. An infusion of the leaves or a poultice was considered useful for all infections and inflammations of the hands and feet, fingers and toes.

Hangover

MAGICO-MEDICINE – The hangover is such an uncomfortable thing to have that all sorts of cures have ben devised, many of which have a basis in Transference Magic. Frogs were again thought to be good recipients of one's self-administered hangover. If one vomited over a frog then threw it as far away as possible, then it was hoped that it would take away the hangover.

Snails too were thought of as worthy of giving one's hangover to. A snail or slug was rubbed over the forehead nine times, then thrown as far away as possible.

Amethysts were considered wonderful stones to prevent hang-overs and stave off drunkenness.

TRADITIONAL REMEDIES – Hops (Humulus lupulus), is a calming, sedative, bitter. It eases digestive inflammations and calms the mood. It is taken as a herbal tea and is almost a specific hangover remedy.

'Hair of the Dog that bit you', is a well known remedy. It is a sympathetic principle related to homoeopathy. A small drink of the offending liquor first thing in the morning may help, although fluids are actually what one really requires. A variant is to take a Prairie Oyster, which consists of one egg yolk, one teaspoon of Worcester Sauce, two dashes of vinegar, salt and pepper to flavour. The egg yolk should be poured into a long glass without breaking, then the other ingredients should be added. The secret is, apparently, to swallow the yolk in one go!

Headache

INVOCATIONS – St Denis, St Stephen.

MAGICO-MEDICINE – The Roman historian Pliny tells us of a grisly headache remedy, which consisted of tightly binding the head with the rope which had been used to hang a man. This remedy, it should be noted, apparently recurred in many European countries including England.

In Ireland and Scotland up until the beginning of this century it was thought that the shroud of a prematurely dead person could cure headaches. A strip had to be cut and bound tightly around the head. This and the previous magico-medical charm were kept in households for this purpose.

In the eighteenth and nineteenth centuries headbands or hat bands made from snake-skin were thought to prevent or cure headaches.

DOCTRINE OF SIGNATURES – an infusion of Self-Heal, drunk by the tablespoonful three times a day will often ease tension headaches.

TRADITIONAL REMEDIES – Feverfew (Chrysanthemum parthenium), a warming herb, also called Nosebleed, is useful for migraine. The flowers made into an infusion and taken as a herbal tea are beneficial twice a day.

Peppermint (Mentha piperita), a warming herb, is a well known general tonic. An infusion as a herbal tea is good for relieving congested headaches.

Self-Heal (Prunella vulgaris), also called All Heal, Sicklewort and Hookweed. An infusion of its flowers, drunk by the tablespoon three times a day seems to settle many types of headache.

WATERS – A Mustard bath for twenty minutes is an old and favoured remedy for headache due to upper respiratory congestion. (PLEASE SEE CHAPTER 6 REGARDING MUSTARD BATHS).

Heartburn

INVOCATIONS – St Timothy of Lystra.

MAGICO-MEDICINE – Wearing an opal next to the skin was said to ease many digestive problems.

TRADITIONAL REMEDIES – Chewing a raw potato is one of the most effective means of relieving this discomfort.

Grated Oak bark (Quercus robur), half an ounce in a pint of boiling water, makes a drink that looks like whisky or brandy. A small glassful daily after food is useful for easing heartburn and stomach acidity. It is traditionally known as *Decoctum Quercus.*

Meadowsweet (Flipendula ulmaria), also known as Queen-of-the-meadows and Lace-Maker's Herb, taken as an infusion of the flowers heads, a handful of flowers to a pint of boiling water. It is excellent for stomach acidity, heartburn and indigestion.

WATERS – *Simple Alkaline Waters, or simple soda waters*, are waters mainly containing sodium bicarbonate. Because of the alkalinity of the waters these were understandably considered beneficial in countering the effects of excess acidity in the body. They were, therefore, recommended for heartburn and stomach problems.

Heart problems

INVOCATIONS – St Valentine and St Teresa of Avila.

MAGICO-MEDICINE – Drinking from a gold goblet was at one time considered excellent for someone with a weak heart. Mother-of-Pearl and quartz crystal vessels were also thought to be healing for the heart.

DOCTRINE OF SIGNATURES – Two tablespoonfuls of Rose petals crushed in a tabletspoonful of honey should be left outside overnight in a glass jar. This is then mixed with a pint of water to form a stock solution. A tablespoon every morning is said to strengthen the heart.

Strawberries eaten throughout the summer are also said to strengthen the heart and calm the individual by 'sweetening the heart.'

TRADITIONAL REMEDIES – Cayenne pepper (Capsicum annum) is used as a tonic for the heart. About a quarter of a teaspoon is taken in a cup of water twice a day for as long as felt necessary. It is an antispasmodic, and was also used in older days at the onset of a heart attack. A pinch was placed directly on the tongue.

Hawthorn (Crataegus monogynova), a warming herb, also called Hagthorn, is generally considered tonic to the heart and circulatory system. The leaf buds when chewed taste like Pepper and Salt, yet another country name. *Extract of Hawthorn* was used in conventional medicine in the earlier twentieth century, and is mentioned by Sir William Osler in his famous textbook, *The Practice of Medicine*, which was the standard text in medical schools for many decades.

An old Yorkshire remedy designed to prevent the Angina producing effect of cold winds, was to sprinkle brown sugar into hot bacon fat (from the bottom of the frying pan) and cover a sheet of brown paper with it. When it was cool it was applied to the chest and left under the vest. The cold winds were thought to be unable to penetrate this.

Fasting and drinking all of one's own urine for nine days was at one time advocated by folk healers.

Hiccups

TRADITIONAL REMEDIES – Holding one's breath as one drinks a glass of water is a well-tried method. A more energetic, but equally well used method is to try drinking water from a glass while standing on one's head.

A half teaspoon of cayenne pepper (Capsicum annum) in a glass of water, sipped slowly is said to be a specific for troublesome hiccups.

Hoarse voice

INVOCATIONS – St Bernardino of Siena.

MAGICO-MEDICINE – Wearing a Turquoise stone is said to alleviate a hoarse voice. A Topaz is also said to help all throat problems.

Gargling with the water from a rain-barrel in which a frog had swam, was considered a fine remedy for a 'croaky' voice in the North of Scotland.

WATERS – Simple steam inhalations may help a hoarse voice.

IMPORTANT NOTE – A hoarse voice can have a serious cause. If the voice goes hoarse and does not improve spontaneously, then a medical opinion should be sought after two weeks.

Hysteria

INVOCATIONS – St Dympna, the patron saint of the insane and those who suffered with nervous problems.

MAGICO-MEDICINE – The full moon is traditionally associated with making people of an hysterical nature subject to mood changes. Wearing silver at the time of the full moon used to be thought to minimise the problem. This was thought to be especially the case if a woman had her period at the time of the full moon. Modern day medical astrologers hold that it is not the moon itself which is important, but the zodiacal position of the moon in relation to one's natal horoscope.

Wearing a Tiger's Eye stone is said to calm an hysterical nature and prevent hypochondriacal behaviour. A sardonyx is also said to be excellent for preventing those of an hysterical nature from becoming hysterical.

Drinking from a silver vessel used to be considered effective in preventing hysteria, or calming an hysterical individual down.

TRADITIONAL REMEDIES – Chamomile (Anthemis nobilis), is an excellent relaxant and sedative, long used in hysterical situations. An infusion of the flowers makes a bitter herbal tea which is made palatable with spearmint, honey or grated liquorice root.

WATERS – *Indifferent Waters or simple thermal springs,* are the waters which contain relatively little in the way of minerals, so that they are almost pure water. They were thought to be especially good for nervous and excitable conditions of the nervous system.

Incontinence

MAGICO-MEDICINE – An old Scottish remedy consisted of putting a frog into a tin with a cupful of the sufferer's urine. The tin and the poor creature were shoved up the chimney, and left for however long it took for the urine to evaporate and the creature to mummify. Its legs were then then detached and ground to a powder and given in a whisky toddy to the incontinence sufferer. The rest of the body was kept as a charm for the future.

Indigestion

INVOCATIONS – St Timothy of Lystra.

MAGICO-MEDICINE – Wearing an opal next to the skin was said to ease many digestive problems.

DOCTRINE OF SIGNATURES – Dandelion or Ginger tea are both effective in easing off this symptom. An alternative with dandelion is to take the dried roots, ground and powdered as a coffee substitute.

TRADITIONAL REMEDIES – Gentian (Gentiana lutea), is a well known bitter, useful for digestive troubles. A Stock can be made by infusing an ounce of the grated root in a pint of boiling water. Two tablespoonfuls three times a day is the usual dosage when needed.

Meadowsweet (Flipendula ulmaria), also known as Queen-of-the-Meadows and Lace-Maker's Herb, taken as an infusion of the flower heads, a handful of flowers to a pint of boiling water. It is excellent for stomach acidity, heartburn and indigestion.

Yellow dock (Rumex crispus), taken as an infusion of the grated root (a teaspoon to a pint of boiling water), in a dose of one tablespoon twice a day, is good for digestive inflammations. It works well as a laxative.

WATERS – *Simple Alkaline Waters, or simple soda waters*, are waters mainly containing sodium bicarbonate. Because of the alkalinity of the waters these were understandably considered beneficial in countering the effects of excess acidity in the body. They were, therefore, recommended for indigestion and stomach problems.

Infected wounds

MAGICO-MEDICINE – Diamond and Pearl are said to increase the body's defences against infections of all sorts.
TRADITIONAL REMEDIES – Linen soaked with the previous days urine was once used in many country areas for infected wounds.

Sphagnum Moss (Sphagnum cymbifolium) has been a favourite remedy from American Frontier Medicine, where it was used by the American Indians. Gypsies also advocated its use, especially when it was soaked in the juice of a herbal antiseptic such as garlic or onion.

Infertility

INVOCATIONS – St Agatha, St Fiacre, St Francis of Paola, St Rita of Cascia.
MAGICO-MEDICINE – Since the days of Ancient Egypt the scarab has been regarded as a fertility symbol. Beetles have been worn as amulets by childless women in different countries over many centuries. Indeed, as a piece of sympathetic magic they have been included in remedies to enhance fertility in Greece, the Mediterranean countries and Britain.

Eagle Stones, thought to have been stones left by eagles in their nests to ensure fertility, were imported in quantity from the East in the 17th and 18th centuries. They were thought to aid fertility, pregnancy and labour when worn about the neck.

Drinking from a goblet fashioned from tortoise shell was at one time considered beneficial to those trying to produce a child.

Knots have been associated with blocked energy for centuries. Couples desperate to conceive used to be advised to make sure that they had no clothes with knots in them. Especially when they went to bed, they should ensure that there were no knots in their nightclothes.

In Somerset, young wives wishing to become pregnant quickly used to be advised to go down to the Maypole after the revellers had retired to their beds. There she was to pull up her skirts and climb to the top of theMaypole where she would tie a garland of freshly cut flowers.

Another interesting remedy involves Transference magic and role play about Robin Hood and Maid Marian (see Chapter 7)
TRADITIONAL REMEDIES – Cayenne pepper (Capsicum annum), a warming herb, is used to enhance fertility. About a quarter of a teaspoon is taken in a cup of water twice a day for as long as felt necessary.

Fennel (Foeniculum vulgara), a warming herb, is useful for enhancing fertility. The leaves can be chewed.

Ginseng (Panax ginseng), while not being considered a fertility herb, is said to be excellent for enhancing the sexual potency of both sexes. As a warming herb it has a rational for stimulating fertility.
WATERS – Both partners should try having a hot Sitz-bath twice or three times a week, adding a handful of lavendar to the hot part. (SEE CHAPTER 6 REGARDING SITZ-BATHS)

Injuries

INVOCATIONS – St Giles.
MAGICO-MEDICINE – Wearing ivory is thought to protect the wearer from sudden injury and accidents.
DOCTRINE OF SIGNATURES – Figwort or Carpenter's Herb *(Poor Man's Salve)* was thought to heal all minor cuts and scratches (which carpenters might sustain). An infusion of the whole herb or a poultice made from the soaked leaves were used.
TRADITIONAL REMEDIES – Comfrey (Symphytum officinale), also called Knitbone and Pigweed, makes an excellent healing ointment for cuts and grazes. A handful of the dried leaves should be pound in a pestle and mortar and mixed with vegetable fat or cold cream. It can be applied several times a day.

Insomnia

MAGICO-MEDICINE – Wearing an amethyst, emerald or sapphire, or going to bed with one under the pillow is said to remove the problem of insomnia.

An old English medical manuscript describes the magical power of Agrimony (Agrimonia Eupatoria) in promoting sleep. A few of the herbs were simply scattered upon the pillow, for:

> 'If it be leyd under mann's heed,
> He shall sleepyn as he were deed;
> He shall never drede ne wakyn
> Till fro under his heed it be takyn.'

DOCTRINE OF SIGNATURES – Nutmeg, grated and sprinkled on hot milk last thing at night was considered a useful hypnotic.

Skullcap also has a very long history for the treatment of insomnia. An infusion can be taken at night, although tablets are available from herbalists and health shops.

IMPORTANT NOTE At the time of writing, however, I feel that this remedy should only be taken under the supervision of a qualified health professional.

Valerian (Valeriana officinalis), also called All Heal (so do not confuse with Self-Heal), St George's Herb and Garden Heliotrope. This is another wonderful relaxant and sleep-inducer. Unfortunately, since it too may have a dubious effect upon the liver, it should only be taken under the supervision of a doctor or herbalist.

Itching

MAGICO-MEDICINE – An amethyst worn next to the skin is said to ease an itching tendency.

DOCTRINE OF SIGNATURES – The Common Stinging Nettle, the whole herb made into a lotion or simply dabbing on an infusion is useful for itching skin problems.

Jaundice

MAGICO-MEDICINE – An old Swedish remedy involved roasting and eating a yellowhammer bird. A less brutal method involved merely showing a yellowhammer to the jaundiced individual:

> *"..if this bird be looked upon by anyone who has the yellow jaundice, the person is cured, but the bird dies."*

> ......but at least it was given a chance to fly away!

Drinking from a gold vessel used to be considered useful for jaundice.

DOCTRINE OF SIGNATURES – Dandelion tea drunk twice or three times a day.

TRADITIONAL REMEDIES – Fasting for nine days and drinking every drop of one's own urine was at one time recommended by folk healers.

Jealousy

MAGICO-MEDICINE – Wearing an emerald or a sardonyx were thought to guard against jealousy.

WATERS – *Indifferent Waters or simple thermal springs,* are the waters which contain relatively little in the way of minerals, so that they are almost pure water. They were thought to be especially good for nervous and excitable conditions of the nervous system.

Joint problems

TRADITIONAL REMEDIES – Cider Vinegar and honey may work well (see ARTHRITIS).

Kidney problems

MAGICO-MEDICINE – The following little incantation was used in by-gone days. It had to be said at the first sign of a urinary problem:

> *"I save myself from this disease of the urine
> ....save us cunnings birds
> ....bird flocks of witches save us."*

Wearing a bloodstone is said to protect against kidney disorders.

DOCTRINE OF SIGNATURES – Burdock root soaked overnight to make an infusion, was thought useful for all urinary problems, especially stones.

TRADITIONAL REMEDIES – Parsley Piert (Alchemilla arvensis), also called Breakstone or Colicwort, taken as an infusion of the whole plant twice a day is useful for soothing the discomfort associated with many bladder and urinary problems.

Parsley (Petroselinum crispum), taken as a daily tisane made from the dried or fresh leaves is a well-established urinary soother and diuretic.

Barley water (Hordeum pratense) is a remedy which is still commonly advised by Family Doctors. A handful of pearl barley is scalded in a pint of water and simmered for twenty minutes. It is then strained and flavoured with lemon juice. A tumblerful three times a day will usually ease the discomfort of many urinary problems.

WATERS – For someone troubled by recurrent kidney infections (provided that the diagnosis has been confirmed), then a Sitz-bath twice a week may help. It will often work particularly well if a handful of chamomille flowers and leaves are added to the hot part of the bath.

(PLEASE SEE CHAPTER 6 REGARDING SITZ-BATHS).

Lameness

INVOCATIONS – St Giles.

MAGICO-MEDICINE – Mice and shrews were thought to carry all sorts of ailments, particularly lameness. Carrying a live shrew in a box or pot about the neck, until it died was a remedy of antiquity which was used to cure lameness, paralysis and apoplexy (strokes).

A mediaeval remedy for lameness was to slaughter a sheep and skin it. The skin was then to be worn against the sufferer's naked flesh for several days.

TRADITIONAL REMEDIES – A very common remedy advocated by Gypsies and country folk in Yorkshire was to mix cow dung in vinegar and boil the mixture. A thick poultice was then wrapped around the swollen part, the poultice being replaced every day or two. It was said to work equally well on horses, cattle and humans.

A related remedy was to mix cow dung in the individual's own urine and boil the mixture. A thick poultice was applied as above. WATERS – For someone particularly troubled by arthritis of the hips or weakness of the lower limbs, a Sitz-bath twice a week might be helpful. It will often work particularly well if a handful of dried nettle leaves are added to the hot part of the bath. (PLEASE SEE CHAPTER 6 REGARDING SITZ-BATHS).

Laryngitis

INVOCATIONS – St Bernardino of Siena.
MAGICO-MEDICINE – Wearing a Turquoise stone is said to alleviate a hoarse voice and prevent laryngitis. A topaz was also said to be beneficial when worn next to the skin.
WATERS – Simple steam inhalations may help a hoarse voice.
IMPORTANT NOTE – A hoarse voice can have a serious cause. If the voice goes hoarse and does not improve spontaneously, then a medical opinion should be sought after two weeks.

Love philtres and charms

MAGICO-MEDICINE – Bezoar Stones, concretions found in the stomachs of ruminant animals all over the world – such as cattle, antelopes, goats and llamas – have been used as ingredients in love potions.

Toadstones, were similar to Adder stones, in that they were hard concretions thought to have come from the heads of very old toads. They were also thought to be important ingredients in love potions.

The bones of a frog or toad have been used by young women since the days of the Romans until quite recent years. It is said that if ants are allowed to eat away the flesh of a dead toad or frog until there is nothing left but the bones, then one has the makings for a powerful love charm that no man can resist. The bones are taken and thrown into a bucket of water. Those which sink should be retrieved and sewn into a small linen bag and worn as a love charm. Apparently, however, if a man should open the bag by some chance, then it would be his hatred and not his love which would follow.

An amber necklace was a traditional gift in Scotland from a mother to her daughter upon the wedding night. It was said to make the bride irrisistable to her husband when they consummated their marriage, and would bind him to her for life.

An old Italian belief was that if a mother gave a prospective son-in-law a piece of her daughter's umbilical cord (kept since her birth) powdered in wine or in a cake, then he would be so overcome with love that he would have to propose marriage to her.

Drinking from Unicorn horn vessels (actually from the tusk of a narwhal) was thought to bind the two drinkers and inflame their passion.

Love problems

INVOCATIONS – St Rita, the patron saint of broken hearts and thwarted desires.
MAGICO-MEDICINE – Wearing Opal is said to sort out a love problem in one's mind – one way or the other.

Madness

INVOCATIONS – St Dympna, the patron saint of the insane and those who suffered with nervous problems.
MAGICO-MEDICINE – A diamond worn next to the skin was said to ease the nerves and help to protect from madness.

Drinking from a silver vessel used to be considered a way of staving off the horrors of madness.
WATERS – *Indifferent Waters or simple thermal springs,* are the waters which contain relatively little in the way of minerals, so that they are almost pure water. They were thought to be especially good for nervous and excitable conditions of the nervous system.

Menopausal problems

MAGICO-MEDICINE – Throughout history people have tried to stave off the effects of ageing. For many women the menopause brought home to them the fact that they were ageing. Any charm or remedy which would halt that event was to be welcomed.

In Antiquity, it was believed that if one could regularly drink human milk one would offset the effects of age.

In Ancient Rome consuming the ovaries of a young animal was thought to imbue the individual with the vitality of youth and would delay the menopause.

Wearing a malachite was thought to ease one through the menopause without problem.

TRADITIONAL REMEDIES – Hawthorn (Crataegus monogynova), a warming herb, also called Hagthorn, is generally considered tonic to the heart and circulatory system. Taken as an infusion twice a day, it may well ease off troublesome hot flushes.

St John's Wort or Balm to the Warrior's Wound, an infusion taken by the tablespoon three times a day is good for lifting the spirits during the menopause.

WATERS – Some people who suffer from troublesome hot flushes may gain relief from a cold Sitz-bath twice or three times a week. (PLEASE SEE CHAPTER 6 REGARDING SITZ-BATHS).

Menstrual problems

MAGICO-MEDICINE – Wearing sapphire and malachite stones were thought to be good for regularising period problems and reducing period pains.

Drinking from a silver vessel used to be recommended to women suffering from period pain or other menstrual disorders.

DOCTRINE OF SIGNATURES – an infusion of either St John's Wort or Shepherd's Purse can be taken a tablespoonful three times a day, to reduce both period pains and the amount of blood loss. An infusion of Self-Heal or Sicklewort, can also be taken to ease period pains.

TRADITIONAL REMEDIES – Feverfew (Chrysanthemum parthenium), also called Nosebleed, is useful for sluggish and painful periods. The flowers made into an infusion and taken as a herbal tea are beneficial twice a day.

Yarrow (Acillea millefolium), also called Bloodwort, Woundwort and Staunch-weed, is a warming herb with a reputation as a wound healer and herb which reduces haemmorhage goes back many centuries. It is well known as a herb which is good for easing sluggish and irregular periods and easing period pains.

Chamomile (Anthemis nobilis), a cooling herb, is an excellent relaxant which eases period pains. An infusion of the flowers makes a bitter herbal tea which is made palatable with spearmint, honey or grated liquorice root.

Self-Heal (Prunella vulgaris), also called All Heal, Sicklewort and Hookweed. An infusion of its flowers, drunk by the tablespoon three times a day seems to relieve period cramps.

WATERS – For someone troubled by painful periods, a Sitz-bath twice a week during the second half of their cycle is to be recommended. It will often work particularly well if a handful of chamomille flowers and leaves are added to the hot part of the bath. (PLEASE SEE CHAPTER 6 REGARDING SITZ-BATHS).

Mouth ulcers

MAGICO-MEDICINE – in country districts of Scotland all sorts of mouth infections and ulcers could be improved by putting a live frog's head in the mouth, then yanking the creature out by its legs and hurling it as far away into a stream or undergrowth as one could. The problem was then transferred to the frog.

TRADITIONAL REMEDIES – Marsh Cudweed (Gnaphalium uliginosum) is a well known herb which when made into an infusion, makes an excellent remedy for mouth ulcers and all painful throat problems. It should be used as a mouth wash or gargle and not swallowed.

Nasal polyps

TRADITIONAL REMEDIES – According to American Frontier Medicine, a snuff made from ground ginger root and cloves, taken twice or three times a day, will shrink nasal polyps.

Nausea

DOCTRINE OF SIGNATURES – Ginger root or Ginger tea (with

honey to make it more palatable) taken sparingly, but frequently seems to ease nause from digestive causes.

TRADITIONAL REMEDIES – Cinnamon (Cinnamonum zeylanicum) is useful for nausea. A quarter of a teaspoon is taken in water twice or three times a day.

Gentian (Gentiana lutea), is a well known bitter, useful for easing nausea. Stock can be made by infusing an ounce of the grated root in a pint of boiling water. Two tablespoonfuls three times a day is the usual dosage when needed.

Spearmint tea (Mentha viridis) taken as often as necessary is a good anti-nausea remedy.

Nerves – see Anxiety, depression, fears

Neuralgia – see Pain

Night cramp – see Cramps

Night terrors

INVOCATIONS – St Bartholomew

MAGICO-MEDICINE – It used to be widely believed in Scotland that one who suffered from night terrors, nightmares, or dreams about the dead, could be cured by attending a wake and having the hand of a corpse placed upon their head.

Wearing an amethyst, emerald or sapphire, or having one under the pillow was said to prevent nightmares or night terrors.

Nosebleeds

DOCTRINE OF SIGNATURES – a tablespoonful of an infusion of the flowers of St John's Wort, three times a day is useful in stopping recurrent nose bleeds. Also, Shepherd's Purse infusion taken the same way, or simply by chewing a handful of the herb can be taken. Either remedy can be soaked on cotton wool and applied directly into the bleeding nostril with good effect, while external compression is given to the nose.

TRADITIONAL REMEDIES – Feverfew (Chrysanthemum parthenium), also called Nosebleed, is useful for recurrent nosebleeds. The flowers made into an infusion and taken as a herbal tea are beneficial twice a day.

According to American Frontier Medicine and an old English country cure, a drop of vinegar placed in the ear on the same side as the bleeding nostril would quickly stop the flow of blood.

Obesity

TRADITIONAL REMEDIES – Fennel (Foeniculum vulgara), a warming herb, is reputed to be helpful in dealing with obesity. The leaves can be chewed.

Celery tisane taken twice a day is a diuretic which may help by initially removing fluid.

Bladderwrack (Fucus vesiculosus), also called Kelp or Popper Sea-Weed is exactly that – common brown seaweed. It should be picked off rocks at low tide and allowed to dry in a warm exposed place. An infusion of it can be taken three times a day for about three or four days at a time. Alternatively, Kelp tablets are available from most health shops. It can be marvellously effective at getting the metabolism balanced. It is as well, however, to take it under the direction of a health professional.

WATERS – A Sitz-bath twice a week is to be recommended, because it may well stimulate the circulation and the metabolism. It is an idea to mix a handful of salt and some Kelp to the hot part of the bath.

(PLEASE SEE CHAPTER 6 REGARDING SITZ-BATHS).

Oedema

MAGICO-MEDICAL – It used to be thought that any herb found growing in a churchyard would be beneficial for the dropsy. Nettles were particular favourites.

TRADITIONAL REMEDIES – Infusions of barley, dandelion, nettle and celery are all mild diuretics which may help mildly swollen ankles or asist with fluid retention. A cup two or three times a day should suffice.

MEDICAL NOTE – In days gone-by the condition of 'Dropsy' was viewed with fear. It may have been caused by liver, kidney or heart disease. In 1775 Sir William Withering, an English physician discovered that a country cure being used by a Folk Medicine practitioner effectively cured a patient (whom he considered incurable) from dropsy. His subsequent experimentation revealed that foxgloves were the active ingredient of the herbal tea. Digitalis, from which we get the modern drug Digoxin, was the result of further investigations over the ensuing years. It is an undoubted life-saver. ONE SHOULD ADD THAT UNDER NO CIRCUMSTANCES SHOULD ONE TRY TO USE FOXGLOVES IN ANY INTERNAL REMEDY. IT IS DANGEROUS IN THE EXTREME.

Pain

DOCTRINE OF SIGNATURES – Elecampane or Horseheal (Wild Sunflower) is useful for muscular aches and pains when the whole herb is added to a bath in which one soaks. St John's Wort or Balm to the Warrior's Wound, an infusion taken by the tablespoon three times a day is good for all manner of acute pains, such as toothache, crushed or trapped fingers, neuralgia, arthritis and painful joints.

TRADITIONAL REMEDIES – According to American Frontier Medicine, painful rheumatic conditions can be eased by making a poultice of soot (one handful), two egg whites and a handful of rose petals. These should be thoroughly mixed together and applied daily to the area.

An alternative Frontier Medicine remedy was to take a handful of bran, a mug of beer, a handful of chamomille flowers and a handful of melliot blossom. These were to be thoroughly mixed together and applied daily to the area.

Palpitations

INVOCATIONS – St Valentine and St Teresa of Avila.
TRADITIONAL REMEDIES – Chamomile (Anthemis nobilis), a

cooling herb, is an excellent relaxant which may prevent palpitations if taken as a tisane twice a day.

IMPORTANT NOTE – Any sudden abnormal heart rhythms may indicate a heart disorder. A medical opinion should be sought in the first instance.

Paralysis

MAGICO-MEDICINE – Mice and shrews were thought to carry all sorts of ailments, particularly lameness. Carrying a live shrew in a box or pot about the neck, until it died was a remedy of antiquity which was used to treat lameness, paralysis and apoplexy (strokes).

Parasites

DOCTRINE OF SIGNATURES – dried Pumpkin seeds crushed in a tablespoon of castor oil and a spoonful of honey, taken after a day's fast were said to get rid of parasitic worms. A few of the sun-dried seeds taken regularly were said to prevent recurrences.

Pleurisy

MAGICO-MEDICINE – An opal worn next to the skin is said to prevent all sorts of lung disorder.

TRADITIONAL REMEDIES – Pleurisy Root (Asclepias tuberosa) is a traditional remedy for pleurisy, a type of chest infection in which the pleura, the covering of the lung, is inflamed. It classically produces pain which is worse on coughing or taking a deep breath. An infusion of the whole herb, a cupful twice a day, may help the discomfort.

IMPORTANT NOTE – Pleurisy is not a condition to self-medicate, because other more serious conditions could be masked. A medical opinion is essential in the first instance.

Poison

INVOCATIONS – St Benedict.

MAGICO-MEDICINE – In days gone-by people had a morbid fear

of poisoning, both accidental and deliberate. The Romans devised many talismans and amulets to protect them from such a death. They have been manufactured to this day as charms to guard against the Evil Eye (see Chapter 2).

The Cross of St Benedict was regarded as a powerful talisman against poisoning. The abreviations on the talisman are in latin, the relevant text being:

> *Sunt mala quae libas,*
> *Ipse venena bibas*

which means

> *What thou offerest is evil*
> *Thou thyself drinkest poison*

Snake bites were also a common fear – (see SNAKEBITES).

Postrate problems

TRADITIONAL REMEDIES – Couch Grass is an old remedy advocated for middle aged men troubled by frequency of passage of urine with dribbling and a tendency to have to get up in the night to urinate. The bruised roots should be boiled in wine, a glass of which is taken in the evening and at bedtime. Care has to be taken in case too much is taken – remembering its laxative action!

Gravel-Root (Eupatorium purpueum), also called Joe Pye Weed, is another traditional remedy for these symptoms. It was used a lot by American Indians and was a favoured herb in Western Frontier Medicine. An ounce of the whole herb in a pint of water should be infused. A wineglassful four or five times a day is said to be very effective for a few days at a time.

WATERS – For someone particularly troubled by the symptoms of prostate trouble, a Sitz-bath twice or three times a week is to be recommended. It will often work particularly well if a handful of chamomille flowers and leaves are added to the hot part of the bath. (PLEASE SEE CHAPTER 6 REGARDING SITZ-BATHS).

IMPORTANT NOTE – Prostate troubles need to be investigated, because cancer of the prostate could be missed by delaying a visit to the doctor. A medical opinion should be sought in the first instance.

Sciatica

MAGICO-MEDICINE – In Devon, sciatica used to be called *boneshave*. To cure it, a sufferer had to go to a river and act out the following little ritual and incantation. While lying beside the river, preferably one flowing Southwards, with a stout stick between him and the river, he had to cry out:–

> *"Boneshave right, boneshave straight,*
> *As the water runs by the stave, good for boneshave."*

TRADITIONAL REMEDIES – Opodeldoc used to be advised. It was rubbed well into the small of the back every four to six hours. (see BACKACHE.)

Cider Vinegar and honey may work well (see ARTHRITIS).

WATERS – For someone particularly troubled by sciatica, a Sitz-bath twice or three times a week is to be recommended. It will often work particularly well if a handful of dried nettle leaves are added to the hot part of the bath.

A Mustard bath is a traditional remedy for sciatica sufferers. While it will not ease genuine sciatica, many cases of muscular leg pain (often called 'sciatica') may improve.
(PLEASE SEE CHAPTER 6 REGARDING MUSTARD AND SITZ-BATHS).

Shingles

INVOCATIONS – St Antony, St Benedict and St John.

MAGICO-MEDICAL – This painful condition was understandably associated with many amulets, talismans and spells. The amulets of St Antony and St Benedict were considered valuable protectives against both this and Erysipelas.

Black cats, being associated in the popular mind with magic were considered to hold a cure for the shingles sufferer. The ear of a black cat was cut off and the blood allowed to drip over the painful part. Then, using some of the blood as ink, the patient's name was written on paper or parchment, then thrown into the fire.

Fortunately for them, Donkeys had a less sacrificial role to play, due to their being regarded as 'holy animals'. The black cross on their backs, reputedly due to having carried Jesus, was thought to be a natural source of healing. Some hair clippings were taken and boiled in water, then painted over the affected area.

IMPORTANT NOTE – Shingles is an extremely painful condition caused by a flare-up of the chickenpox virus within a skin nerve. It is not something which you catch, but something which has been dormant since you had chickenpox.

In days when Erysipelas was common it is not surprising that it would be confused with Shingles and the two conditions treated in the same way.

Sinusitis

TRADITIONAL REMEDIES – According to American Frontier Medicine, sinusitis could be treated by scraping carrots and softening them on a fire shovel. If they were then applied over the tender cheekbones they eased the pain and helped to reduce the inflammation. This was regarded as a good way of soothing many inflammatory conditions. (see BREAST PROBLEMS, EYE PROBLEMS).

WATERS – A Mustard foot bath for twenty minutes is an old and favoured remedy for helping with colds and sinusitis.

(PLEASE SEE CHAPTER 6 REGARDING MUSTARD BATHS).

Skin problems

DOCTRINE OF SIGNATURES – The Common Stinging Nettle, the whole herb made into a lotion or an infusion dabbed over the area is useful for all itching and burning skin conditions. .

TRADITIONAL REMEDIES – Romany Balm (see Absesses and boils above) was advocated by Gypsies.

WATERS – Oat baths twice a week are very useful for very

irritated skin problems. Three or four goods handfuls of oats are traditionally wrapped in a tea-towel and infused in a warm bath.

Sulphated waters containing Epsom salts are traditionally used for conditions like psoriasis. Two handfuls of Epsom salts in a warm bath two or three times a week will often help the psoriasis sufferer. Only a bath of ten minutes should be used. (see CHAPTER 6 re OAT AND EPSOM BATHS).

Snake bites

INVOCATIONS – St Hilary, St Blaise, St Patrick, St Vitus
MAGICO-MEDICINE – an amulet made from the leaf of the Greater Plantain or Snakeweed, was considered a protection against snakebite.

The following ritual and incantation were considered useful for Adder bites. Two pieces of hazel wood had to be placed across the bite in the shape of a cross while the following incantation was sung:–

> *"Underneath this hazelin mote,*
> *There's a maggoty worm with a speckled throat.*
> *Nine double is he;.*
> *And from nine double to eight double,*
> *And from eight double to seven double.........*

and continuing until:–

> *And from One double to no double,*
> *No double hath he."*

And this was supposed to reduce the swelling and reduce any effect of the poison.

Agates are traditional stones which are said to prevent snake-bites. They are also said to absorb the poison if rubbed against the bite wound.
DOCTRINE OF SIGNATURES – Green Oil of Charity (Adder's Tongue) applied night and morning to the wound.

In the highland moors of Scotland, where adders were common, so-called *Adder stones* were eagerly sought after. These were thought to have been produced by the concretion of adder spit. Small Adder stones were believed to be effective against snake-bites, eye problems and the whooping cough in children.

Sore throat

INVOCATIONS – St Andrew, St Blaise

MAGICO-MEDICINE – The Roman historian Pliny reports that throat diseases and glandular trouble would be cured if the hand of a corpse was placed on the troubled part. To be most effective, it was thought that the corpse had to be that of someone who had died prematurely.

Ever since the 16th century, sore throat sufferers have been invited to take the blessing of St Blaise. This involves placing two candles upon the throat, since the saint is always portrayed as holding two candles.

Wearing a Topaz is said to protect one from throat infections and to quickly speed them on their way.

TRADITIONAL REMEDIES – At one time people used to tie a red thread about their neck whenever afflicted with a sore throat.

A related remedy consisted of tying a several days old sock around the neck when one went to bed. This is a remedy which is still much used today.

Marsh Cudweed (Gnaphalium uliginosum) is a well known herb which when made into an infusion, makes an excellent remedy for mouth ulcers and all painful throat problems. It should be used as a mouth wash or gargle and not swallowed.

Self-Heal (Prunella vulgaris), also called All Heal, Sicklewort and Hookweed. An infusion of its flowers, drunk by the tablespoon three times a day seems to ease sore throats.

Coltsfoot (Tussilago farfara), also known as Coughwort is perhaps one of the best known traditional cough mixtures. It is also extremely good if taken as a gargle and remedy for sore throat. A handful of the flowers should be infused in a pint of water and left to cool. A glass or cupful, sweeted with liquorice root or melted honey three times a day will often soothe a painful throat. Gargling with the remedy will often soothe the pain of the throat. A Sage gargle is also quite excellent for easing a sore throat.

Sprains

MAGICO-MEDICINE – An old magico-medical remedy consists of tying a string or cord around the sprained part. As one does this one ties nine knots. The knots are then untied as the following incantation is made:

> 'I knot the string nine times over,
> I untie each one once.
> Yet one is nine and nine is one,
> When that one is gone I will recover.'

TRADITIONAL REMEDIES – Opodeldoc used to be advised, provided there was no breakage of the skin (See BACKACHE).
WATERS – For sprained ankles a mustard foot bath alternating with a cold footbath is a traditional remedy.

Stammering

INVOCATIONS – St Bartholomew.
MAGICO-MEDICINE – Eating roast nightingale is a traditional remedy for curing the problem of stammering.

Wearing a Turquoise stone is said to help to keep the problem under control.

TRADITIONAL REMEDIES – According to legend, a great Greek philosopher and orator cured himself of a difficult stammer by placing a pebble in his mouth and trying to shout above the noise of the waves.

Stings

MAGICO-MEDICINE – The best known Folk cure of all is the use of a Dock leaf to cure the sting of a nettle. To work best, however, it is said to require an incantation as well. There are several variants, but this one has a considerable antiquity:–

> *Nettle in, dok out, now this, now that."*

Geoffrey Chaucer (14th century)

In my country the alternative one has apparently been used for centuries.

> *In dockin leaf, nettle leave alain (alone).*

If stung by a bee or wasp, the injured party was advised to catch the insect if possible and drown it in a bottle with one's own urine. The urine was thought to neutralise the creature's poison, so that if the urine was then rubbed over the injured part, it would take the pain away!

DOCTRINE OF SIGNATURES – Green Oil of Charity (Adder's Tongue) applied night and morning to the sting.

TRADITIONAL REMEDIES – Ant and horsefly bites can be eased by rubbing a raw onion over the wound.

Bee stings might be soothed by dabbing the wound with bicarbonate of soda solution, after removing the sting with a small forceps.

Midge bites can be eased by bruising a dock leaf or a sage leaf and rubbing over the area.

Stomach

INVOCATIONS – St Timothy of Lystra.

MAGICO-MEDICINE – An opal worn next to the skin is said to ease all sorts of digestive problem.

Drinking from crystal used to be considered beneficial to the stomach.

DOCTRINE OF SIGNATURES – Liquorice root, chewed directly or taken in an infusion with honey is excellent for soothing stomach problems or helping with the pain of an ulcer. An infusion of Self-Heal, taken by the tablespoonful three times a day will often ease the pains of stomach ulceration.

TRADITIONAL REMEDIES – Meadowsweet (Flipendula ulmaria), also known as Queen-of-the-meadows and Lace-Maker's Herb, taken as an infusion of the flowers heads, a handful of flowers to a pint of boiling water. It is excellent for stomach acidity, heartburn and indigestion.

Styes

MAGICO-MEDICINE – It used to be said that if a stye was rubbed nine times with the tail of a black cat, the stye would go by the following morning.

Rubbing a stye with an emerald is also said to work.

DOCTRINE OF SIGNATURES – a lotion of Euphrasia, applied four times a day will often relieve a painful stye.

TRADITIONAL REMEDIES – Fresh garden dew bottled and rubbed over the stye two or three times a day is an old Scottish remedy for all sorts of eye and eyelid problems. A gold wedding ring rubbed over the stye is a commonly used Folk practice to this day. Similarly, a piece of amber rubbed over a stye was said to cause the stye to shrivel and resolve. From memory I remember the amber mouthpiece of a meerschaum pipe being used.

Sunburn

TRADITIONAL REMEDIES – Potato juice is a very old country remedy which may be safely applied to a small area of sunburn. The cut surface of the potato is gently rubbed over the area and repeated when necessary.

Stawberries are also useful. Two or three are crushed and the juice smeared over the area. It is left on for half an hour or so, then washed off. It can be repeated as often as necessary.

Cider vinegar also has a reputation of easing the pain in mild sunburn. It should be noted, however, that it will sting for a few minutes, before it begins to soothe the area.

Thrush

MAGICO-MEDICINE – in country districts of Scotland all

sorts of mouth infections and ulcers could be improved by putting a live frog's head in the mouth, then yanking the creature out by its legs and hurling it as far away into a stream or undergrowth as one could. The problem was then transferred to the frog.

TRADITIONAL REMEDIES – Chewing a clove of garlic, although seeming anti-social will often remove the problem of oral and intestinal thrush. It can also be highly effective in getting rid of vaginal thrush.

Live yoghurt, a good sized portion eaten once a day will often clear up resistant thrush, especially if a little is used as a cream on the affected parts three times a day.

Thyroid problems

MAGICO-MEDICINE – Goitres were the usual problem complained of in Folk Medicine. They were referred to as Wens, and were often treated by Transference Magic. One such remedy involved stroking the throat with a live snake nine times, then burying the snake alive in a bottle. As it died and decomposed, so it was thought that the goitre would go away.

It was commonly believed up until this century that the hand of a corpse could cure a wen, or thyroid goitre. People with goitres would accordingly attend a wake in order to have the corpse's hand placed upon their goitre.

Wearing a Blue Tourmaline stone is thought to be excellent for helping a thyroid problem.

TRADITIONAL REMEDIES – Bladderwrack (Fucus vesiculosus), also called Kelp or Popper Sea-Weed tablets are said to have a beneficial effect upon the thyroid gland. Stimulating an underactive gland and sedating it when it is overactive. It is not one for self treatment, however. It should be taken under the advice of a health professional.

Tics and twitches

INVOCATIONS – St Bartholomew, St Cornelius.
MAGICO-MEDICINE – The comb from a rooster worn as an

amulet was considered helpful in days gone-by, since hens move their heads in rapid twitch-like movements.

TRADITIONAL REMEDIES – Mugwort soaked in water overnight and used for washing the hands was advocated in American Frontier Medicine.

Tinnitus

MAGICO-MEDICINE – Wearing a small bell was a common amulet to ward off the Evil Eye. The sound of the bell, being 'sympathetic' to the noise of tinnitus may have made it a suitable charm for this distressing condition.

TRADITIONAL REMEDIES – In past days folk healers advised instilling warm urine in the ears.

Toothache

INVOCATIONS – St Elizabeth of Hungary, St Apollonia.

MAGICO-MEDICINE – In country areas it was recommended that the gum overlying the tooth should be scratched with a nail or jagged piece of wood found in a graveyard. The nail should then be hammered into a tree or the wood buried in an old grave. The toothache would be transferred from the sufferer.

The foot of a mole, if cut off while the poor animal was still living, was used in many parts of England in olden times as a cure for toothache when worn as an amulet. The Romans also advocated attaching the tooth from a mole to one's clothing.

Wearing a malachite stone is thought to be protective against toothache. Rubbing the gum overlying the troublesome tooth is also said to ease the pain.

DOCTRINE OF SIGNATURES – The acute pain of toothache may be relieved by taking a tablespoonful of an infusion of St John's Wort three times a day (or more frequently until the dentist is seen).

TRADITIONAL REMEDIES – Tincture of Myrrh applied to the painful area will often relieve toothache.

Travel sickness

INVOCATIONS – St Christopher.

MAGICO-MEDICINE – Consuming a meal made from a creature known to be a 'traveller' was said to avert travel sickness. Pigeon pie or jellied eels were both advocated.

TRADITIONAL REMEDIES – Chewing a little ginger root before travelling is often quite effective.

Ulcers of the skin

DOCTRINE OF SIGNATURES – Green Oil of Charity (Adder's Tongue) applied daily to the ulcer. Oil of St John's Wort applied in the same way is also effective.

TRADITIONAL REMEDIES – Self-Heal (Prunella vulgaris), also called All Heal, Sicklewort and Hookweed. An infusion of its flowers, drunk by the tablespoon three times a day seems to promote healing of wounds and ulcers.

Urinary infections

MAGICO-MEDICINE – The following little incantation was used in by-gone days. It had to be said at the first sign of a urinary problem:

> *"I save myself from this disease of the urine*
> *....save us cunnings birds*
> *....bird flocks of witches save us."*

DOCTRINE OF SIGNATURES – Burdock root soaked overnight to make an infusion was thought to be valuable for all urinary infections. A cup or glass was taken twice a day.

TRADITIONAL REMEDIES – Horse-radish (Cochlearia armoracia), a warming herb, is used as a remedy to relieve urinary tract infections. One or two roots, grated down and taken daily in several divided doses before meals. Taking bread at the same time will reduce the heat in one's mouth.

Varicose veins

TRADITIONAL REMEDIES – Peppermint (Mentha piperita), a warming herb, is good for easing the pains of varicose veins. An infusion as a herbal tea is taken twice a day.

Cayenne pepper (Capsicum annum), a warming remedy is useful for aching varicose veins. About a quarter of a teaspoon is taken in a cup of water twice a day for as long as felt necessary.

A sage bath is also an excellent restorative for aching legs secondary to varicose veins.

WATERS – A Mustard bath for twenty minutes is an old and favoured remedy for aching legs secondary to varicose veins. (PLEASE SEE CHAPTER 6 REGARDING MUSTARD BATHS).

Vitality

MAGICO-MEDICINE – It is said that if one wears a turquoise stone, it will show your state of health. When ill, it will go dull and pale. As one's vitality increases, it regains its colour.

Drinking from a goblet fashioned from tortoise shell was at one time considered a good tonic in itself, because of the age that the tortoise could live to.

Warts

MAGICO-MEDICINE – Culpepper recommended rubbing a wart with a live snail nine times, then impaling the creature upon a blackthorn. As it died, so would the wart disappear.

It was commonly believed up until this century that the hand of a corpse could remove a wart or growth. Accordingly, people used to attend wakes in order to achieve a cure by lifting the corpse's hand onto their warts.

My grandfather told me of a sure-fire wart cure when I was young. One had to count the number of warts one had, then get a piece of string and tie that number of knots in it. Each wart had to be touched with a knot. The string was then taken and hurled into a stagnant pool or ditch where it would rot away. And as it rotted, so would the warts disappear.

Mark Twain has his famous character Tom Sawyer recite a wart cure which was obviously used on the banks of the Mississippi. It consisted of cutting a bean in half and rubbing both halves over the wart. One half was to be burned and the other buried at a cross-roads.

TRADITIONAL REMEDIES – My mother told me of the following Folk remedies for warts. Cabbage water drained from boiled cabbage and allowed to cool was to be applied daily for as long as it took the wart to go white and craggy in appearance. Potato water was also used.

A small square of banana skin is cut and applied to the surface of the wart (after the wart had been roughened with a pummice stone), the pith side of the skin to the wart. This was taped onto the skin and left overnight. Upon its removal the wart will be black. This is repeated nightly until the wart resolves.

According to American Frontier Medicine, warts can be cured by mixing brown soap with saliva and applying directly to the wart. If this is left for twenty-four hours then the wart will come away as the hardened soap is peeled away.

Yet another Frontier remedy consisted of taking the lung of a newly slaughtered sheep and letting the blood run out of it. Then, the lung was pressed to squeeze out remaining fluid. This was collected in a bottle and dabbed on warts as and when they appeared. It was said to be a wonderous remedy.

Celandine, Greater (Chelidonium majus), is a herb which can be poisonous internally and corrosive when applied to the skin. It is the latter property which added its name to Folk Medicine, where it became known as – *Wartwort*.

Water retention – see Oedema

TRADITIONAL REMEDIES – Infusions of barley, dandelion, nettle, parsley and celery are all mild diuretics which may help mildly swollen ankles or assist with fluid retention. A cup two or three times a day should suffice.

Worms

DOCTRINE OF SIGNATURES – A tablespoonful of dried Pumpkin

seeds crushed in a tablespoonful of castor oil and a spoonful of honey, taken in the morning after a day's fast are said to get rid of worms (tapeworms actually, which are not really a problem, but also the threadworms which are the commonest nematode infestation in developed countries). A few of the sun-dried seeds chewed occasionally are said to prevent recurrence.

TRADITIONAL REMEDIES – Horse-radish (Cochlearia armoracia), a warming herb, is used to expel woms and parasites. One or two roots, grated down and taken daily in several divided doses before meals. Taking bread at the same time will reduce the heat in one's mouth.

Wounds

MAGICO-MEDICINE – In the Middle Ages St Blaise, the patron saint of wool-combers, was often invoked when one had been wounded by a thorn, the tooth of a comb or a splinter. One simply covered the wound with a hand and said:–

> *'Blaise, the martyr, commands thee to come forth,*
> *In the Name of the Lord Jesus Christ.'*

Snake-skins were also used throughout the country as cures for all sorts of puncturing wounds. They were considered a specific remedy for thorn wounds.

DOCTRINE OF SIGNATURES – Oil of St John's Wort, prepared from the finely chopped flowers simmered in oil, is effective in healing puncture wounds, cuts and abrasions. A tablespoonful of an infusion three times a day helps with the associated pain.

TRADITIONAL REMEDIES – Figwort (Scrophularia nodosa), also called the Scrophula Plant, Brownwort, Carpenter's Herb and Poor Man's Salve, is used as an ointment for wounds and sores. The whole herb or leaves boiled in water or oil, made a useful mode of treatment. Alternatively, the soaked leaves can be used as a poultice.

Self-Heal (Prunella vulgaris), also called All Heal, Sicklewort and Hookweed. An infusion of its flowers, drunk by the tablespoon three times a day seems to promote healing of wounds.

Cabbage (Brassica oleracea bullata), shredded and made into a poultice is an excellent wound healer. The poultice needs to be replaced daily and may need to be repeated for weeks in resistant cases. It is, however, a marvellous remedy.

The Saints

As we have seen throughout this book it was common practice throughout the centuries to invoke the name of particular saints when someone was afflicted with particular illnesses. The reason for the association with those ailments or illnesses is often given in the manner of their death, martyrdom, or legends which sprang up around their cult.

St AGNES – the patron saint of couples and virgins. This young Roman girl was martyred by beheading for her Christian beliefs in the early fourth century. She had been sent to a brothel to make her lose her innocence, yet remained pure.

St ALBAN – a pagan soldier of the time of Diocletian. He saved a priest and was converted to Christianity. He was the first British martyr.

St AMAND – the patron saint of brewers, drinkers and barmen. This French Abbot died of natural causes in 679 AD. He travelled throughout the wine-growing areas of France, converting pagans to his religion.

St ANDREW – the patron saint of Scotland, old maids and carer of sore throats and gout. Andrew was a fisherman, one of the disciples. He died in about 60AD, his relics reputedly being taken to a site in Scotland by St Rule. Later a church was built on the site. This town was to become St Andrews.

St ANTONY – the patron saint of basket-makers, and protector against ergotism – St Antony's Fire, erysipelas and epilepsy. This saint was known as 'the Hermit.' He was the founder of monasticism. He died as he wished, in a cave in 356 AD. His emblem is the T-shaped cross which is a well-known charm.

St APOLLONIA – the patron saint of dentists, and protector against toothache. Apollonia, a deaconess, was struck in the face, sustaining a broken jaw and loss of her teeth during riots in Alexandria in 249 AD. She was offered clemency if she renounced her faith, but chose to throw herself onto the execution pyre.

St BARTHOLOMEW – the patron saint of Florence, tanners and leather-workers, and the protector against nervous diseases, stammering and twitching. He was martyred in the first century by being flayed alive then beheaded.

St BENEDICT – the patron saint of Europe and schoolchidren. He was also the protector against fevers and poisoning. He was the founder of the Benedictine order. He died naturally in 545 AD.

St BERNARDINO of SIENA – the patron saint of preachers, and the protector against hoarse voices. A Franciscan monk who pilgrimaged throughout Italy, preaching as he went. He died naturally in 1444 AD.

St BLAISE – the patron saint of wool-combers, and the protector of throat diseases and all puncture wounds. There is a legend that St Blaise healed a boy who was choking to death, hence his association with throat disorders. Living in a cave, tending to the needs of injured wild animals, he was dragged before the Governor of Cappadocia and subsequently tortured with iron wool-combs before being beheaded in 315 AD.

St BRIGID – the second patron saint of Ireland (after St Patrick). She was also the patron saint of blacksmiths, midwives, healers, newborn children and maids. An historical Brigid founded the first convent in Ireland at Kildare, where she died of natural causes in 525 AD. She has been identified with the Celtic goddess Brigid.

St CATHERINE OF ALEXANDRIA – the patron saint of librarians, young girls and spinners. This saint was martyred in 310 AD after she had been subjected to torture with a spiked wheel, 'to break her.' The wheel broke, however, and she was subsequently beheaded.

St CHRISTOPHER – the patron saint of travellers. This saint was said to be a giant of a man. He is said to have transported travellers across a great river by carrying them on his back. One legend says that he once carried a child who was revealed to be Christ. Planting his staff in the ground, it immediately blossomed. He is thought to have been martyred in Asia Minor in the third century.

St CORNELIUS – the patron saint of domestic animals and the protector against earche, epilepsy and nervous twitches. This saint was an early pope who is reputed to have had a liberal attitude towards repentant sinners. He is said to have died in exile in about 250 AD.

St DENIS – the patron saint of France and the protector against headaches. He was said to have been martyred in Paris in 250 AD. According to legend and religious paintings he actually carried his own head to his grave after he had been beheaded.

St DUNSTAN – the patron saint of goldsmiths and jewellers, and the protector of the blind. A Benedictine monk who became Archbishop of Canterbury, he was a powerful reformer of monasticism in Britain. He died at Canterbury in 988 AD.

St DYMPNA – the patron saint of the insane and the mentally ill. Dympna was reputedly a Celtic princess who was murdered by her insane father in the ninth century.

St ELIZABETH of HUNGARY – the patron saint of bakers, beggars and lace-makers. She was a protector against toothache.

Once a queen of Hungary, Elizabeth was exiled after her husband died while on a Crusade. In exile she worked with the needy, tending to their ills and mending clothes. Possibly due to the harsh conditions she lived under, her constitution failed and she died in 1231 AD.

St ERASMUS, also known as St ELMO – the patron saint of sailors. He was also the protector of women in labour and those suffering from colic pains. A legend says that during his martyrdom in 300 AD, he was disembowelled while still living. His fame as a preacher was such that he would preach and people would listen even at the height of a storm. His name is thence also given for the peculiar phosphorescent electrical discharge seen at the top of ships masts after storms – St Elmo's lights.

St FIACRE – the patron saint of gardeners and florists. He was also the protector of those with anal problems and haemorrhoids. An Irish monk, he travelled and preached in France where he also developed great skills in gardening. He is said to have ploughed the soil using only his staff. He died in about 670 AD.

St FRANCIS of PAOLA – the patron saint of sailors. He was often invoked by childless couples. Legend has it that he had to cross the Straits of Messina, so rolled out his cape and attached an end to his staff and sailed across the water. Originally living as a hermit at Paola, he later formed an Order. He died of natural causes in 1507 AD.

St GENEVIEVE – the patron saint of Paris, was also a protector of fever cases. Legend says that she would go to church at night and resist the attempts of the devil to blow out her candle. She died in about 500 AD. Her association with fevers relates to an outbreak of plague in the 12th Century which was stopped when her relics were taken on procession through the city of Paris.

St GILES – The patron saint of beggars and cripples. Legend tells that when this saint was a hermit he lived on the milk from a deer. A hunting party chased this deer into the woods and shot an arrow at it. When they crashed through the undergrowth after it they found that they had wounded St Giles. In fact he was protecting the wounded creature. He died in the early 8th Century.

St GREGORY – the patron saint of singers and musicians. He was a protector against gout. According to the Venerable Bede, Gregory saw some slaves being sold in the Forum at Rome. Upon asking who they were, he was told that they were Angles. He replied that they were not Angles, but *Angles*. He became Pope and died in Rome in 604 AD.

St HILARY of POITIERS – the patron saint of backward children and the protector against snakebites. He died in Poitiers in 350 AD.

St JOHN THE BAPTIST – the patron saint of farriers, tailors, spas and Knights Hospitallers. He became famous for baptising those who came to listen to his preachings. Christ himself came for baptism. He was martyred when Salome asked Herod for 'the head of the Baptist on a platter' after she danced for him.

St MARGARET of ANTIOCH – the patron saint of women. She was also one of the protectors of childbirth. At one time a shepherdess, she was tortured with fire during the persecutions in the time of Diocletian. She was ultimately beheaded and buried at Antioch at the end of the 3rd Century. A legend talks of her being swallowed by a dragon, but escaping by cutting her way out of the creature's abdomen.

St PANCRAS – the patron saint of children and a protecor against cramps. He was martyred at the age of 14 years during the persecutions in the time of Diocletian at the end of the 3rd Century.

St PATRICK – the patron saint of Ireland and the protector against snakes. Legend says that the saint expelled all the snakes from Ireland. He died round about 450 AD.

St RITA of CASCIA – the patron saint of desperate causes. She was often invoked by childless couples. This saint was said to have been born to very aged parents, hence her association with childless couples – there is always hope. She was said to have stigmata on her forehead, like the wounds suffered by Christ from the crown of thorns. She died in Cascia in about 1450 AD.

St STEPHEN – the patron saint of deacons. He was invoked against headaches. At his trial, in about 30 AD, Stephen told his persecutors that he saw Christ standing at the right hand of God. This incensed the persecutors who ordered that he be taken out and stoned to death.

St TERESA OF AVILA – the patron saint of lace-makers. She was a Carmelite nun who died in about 1580. She is portrayed in art with a fiery arrow piercing her heart.

St THOMAS – the patron saint of architects. He was often invoked for eye disorders. Thomas was, of course the original 'doubting Thomas' who would not believe his eyes. He was martyred by being stabbed with a spear sometime during the 1st century.

St TIMOTHY OF LYSTRA – the saint who was advised to 'take a little wine for the stomach.' He was martyred in the 1st century by being stoned to death at Ephesus.

St VALENTINE – the patron saint of lovers. The actual connection with the historical St Valentine, who was martyred in Rome in the 3rd Century, seems very tenuous. The fact is that in Roman times there was a feast called Lupercalia, which was celebrated in the middle of February.

St VITUS – the patron saint of nervous disorders, and of actors and dancers. He was invoked against St Vitus' Dance and against snakebites. He was martyred at the time of Diocletian round about 300 AD.

The Herbs

Here follows a short thumb-nail description of the herbs cited throughout this book. I include here the common name and the usual botanical name. But please again remember that we have a duty to the environment, so these plants should not be plucked from their habitat. Apart from the risks of misidentifying a simple plant for a potentially toxic one, it is far easier to obtain stocks from a reputable supplier. You will find that most will be able to advise you about setting up and maintaining your own herb garden.

Adder's Tongue (Ophioglossum vulgatum), is a small fern with small oval leaves which has a flowering part which resembles an adder's tongue.

Agrimony (Agrimonia Eupatoria) is found in hedgerows and waste land. It has small yellow flowers which taper upwards. The leaves resemble small rose leaves. Usually, it has a smell similar to apricots.

Arnica (Arnica montana) is a mountain plant growing to about two feet in height. The leaves form a flat rosette in the centre of which the orange or yellow flower shoots.

Aspen (Populus tremula) is a British tree found in moist soils. The leaves tremble in even the slightest of winds. There is an old tradition in Scotland that the leaves are never still because the cross was made of Aspen wood.

Basil (Ocimum basilicum) is a useful medicinal and culinary plant with shiny oval leaves. It throws of attractive little white whorl shaped flowers. It grows to about three feet.

Betony (Stachys Betonica), also called Bishopswort, Wood Betony and Sentinel of the Woods. It is a wild plant with a two foot stem and dark red or purple two-lipped flowers growing in whorls.

Birthwort (Aristolochia longa), a herb introduced to England and once grown in monastery gardens. It is not a safe plant and was mentioned for interest only

Bladderwrack (Fucus vesiculosus), also called Kelp or Popper Sea-Weed. It is quite distinctive as the common brown seaweed found on half-covered rocks at the seaside. It has long dangling fronds with bean sized bladders which keep the plant afloat.

Burdock (Arctium lappa), also called *Love Leaves and Clot-bur*, is a distinctive plant with wavy leaves and large purple flowers which grows around old ruins. Its small burs attach themselves to passing animals, thence disseminating the plant widely.

Calamint (Calamintha officinalis), also known as *Bruisewort*, is a green herb which grows along the banks of streams. It is bushy and rarely grows taller than a foot. It has brown hairy leaves arranged in opposing pairs. The pale flowers are indistinct. Its green juice was thought to look like bile, hence its use in gall bladder disease and disorders of the 'spleen.'

Castor Oil Plant (Ricinus communis), also called *Christ's Hand*, was used by the Egyptians and is described in the Ebers Papyrus of about 1550 BC. It grows in tropical, sub-tropical and temperate zones in the world. Its oil has been a valuable commodity for many centuries. Its hand-shaped leaves indicate its general healing content.

Catmint (Nepeta cataria), also called *Catwort or Cat's Delight*, is well known to attract cats. It grows to about two or three feet in height. Its leaves are heart shaped with a slight serrated edge. They also have a velvety hairiness. The lavendar blue flowers grow on long dangling spikes.

Cayenne pepper (Capsicum annum) was introduced into Britain from India in 1548. It is a perrenial shrub growing anything between two and six feet tall. The pepper is readily available over the counter.

Celandine, Greater (Chelidonium majus), used to be used in jaundiced conditions, because of the bright yellow juice which was extractable from it. It was also known as *Swallow-wort, Devil's Milk and Witchwort,* indicating its use in protecting against evil spirits. It is a herb which can be poisonous internally and corrosive when applied to the skin, even although it does have a use when touched on a wart – hence yet another name – *Wartwort*.

Celandine, Lesser (Ranunculus ficaria), also known as *Pilewort*, was used as a topical remedy for varicose veins, haemorrhoids or piles, or as a general poultice. The whole herb was scalded in boiling water or oil, then applied when cool night and morning. The sign leading to its use was the shape of its knobbly roots, which resembled prolapsed piles.

Celery (Apium graveolens) – is quite distinctive with its long brittle, water filled stems.

Chamomile (Anthemis nobilis), was known to the Ancient Egyptians as a cure for ague and dedicated to their Gods Thoth and Imhotep. It grows in fields and waste ground. It sometimes forms a sea of flowers along country walks. It has low feathery, wispy leaves and a distinctive smell. There are single or double headed flowers. It is best to buy the herbs from a supplier rather than trying to identify it oneself.

Cinnamon (Cinnamonum zeylanicum) the wonderful odour of this woody spice is unmistakable.

Coltsfoot (Tussilago farfara), is a creeping herb with big lovely heart shaped leaves, sometimes eight to ten inches across, which give the plant its name. The flowers look like small dandelions.

Comfrey (Symphitum officinale) grows in meadows and damp areas and can be grown in your own herb garden. Its great value is as an ointment. It has a large leafy stem covered with hairs. The leaves are up to ten inches in length and are also hairy. Its throws off drooping yellow or purple flowers. If you do attempt to make an ointment from this plant, a word of warning. It smells if you do not prepare it quickly!

Cuckoo-pint (Arum maculatum), is a distinctive plant also known as *Lords and Ladies*. It is found in shady hedgerows in the spring and summer, its phallic-like flower giving the sign of its use as a potent aphrodisiac. The name is derived from the Anglo-Saxon *cucu*, meaning lively, and *pintle*, meaning penis. IT IS HIGHLY POISONOUS WHILE FLOWERING, SO I MENTION IT MERELY FROM ITS HISTORIC INTEREST.

Couch grass (Agropyron repens), also called *Twitch grass, Dog grass, Dog tooth*, is another example of a plant that dogs and cats instinctively chew when their stomachs are upset. It is the spindley grass weed which is the bane of most gardener's lives. It nuisance value is, however, made up for by its usefulness medicinally.

Dandelion (Taraxacum officinale), also called *Devil's milk-pail,* This plant needs little description. It grows on grassland, waysides and in hedgerows. Its yellow flowers are as distinctive as are the dandelion clocks so beloved of children.

Elecampane (Inula helenium), *the Wild Sunflower, or Horseheal*, was imported to England by returning crusaders. It had apparently been used by the Saracens to deal with muscular injuries and respiratory ailments of their horses.It is a huge wild plant with coarse leaves and big flowers like daisies.

Eyebright (Euphrasia officinalis), also called *Clear-eye,* is a small plant with red or purple and white flowers, spotted with yellow 'eyes'. It should never be taken internally, except in homoeopathic dilutions.

Fennel (Foeniculum vulgara), can be grown in your own herb garden. It can grow very tall if allowed. It has lots of feathery, wispy leaves and yellow florets.

Feverfew (Chrysanthemum parthenium), also called *Nosebleed,* grows on waste areas. It also has feathery leaves with small daisy-like flowers.

Figwort (Scrophularia nodosa), also called the *Scrofula Plant, Brownwort, Carpenter's Herb and Poor Man's Salve,* grows in ditches and damp places. Its flowers are brown wierd cup-shaped. It is beloved by wasps.

Foxglove (Digitalis purpurea), also known *as Witches' Gloves, Bloody Fingers and Dead Man's Thimbles* is well known as the plant from which the heart drug Digitalis and its derivative Digoxin were first prepared. IT IS HIGHLY POISONOUS WHILE FLOWERING, SO I MENTION IT MERELY FROM ITS HISTORIC INTEREST.

Garlic (Allium sativum), also known as *Gypsy's Onions,* has a distinctive appearance and odour.

Gentian (Gentiana lutea), grows in damp areas, marshlands and around water. It grows to about four feet and has greenish yellow oblong, pointed leaves with orange-yellow flowers in clusters. It is quite a woody herb.

Ginger (Zingiber officinale) is a well known plant and spice, the convolutions of its rhizome resembling the appearance of the bowel.

Ginseng (Panax ginseng), grows to about three feet in height, depending upon its age. It has serrated leaves and produces pale green flowers after a few years. The underground root is the distinctive feature of this plant. It is available from most health shops and chemists.

Gravel-Root (Eupatorium purpueum), also called Joe Pye Weed, comes from America and Canada, where it grows in swampy areas to a height of about six feet. It has a long purple stem with oblong leaves. Its flowers are also purple.

Hawthorn (Crataegus monogynova), also called Hagthorn, is a British tree with dark green narrow leaves. It is common in English hedgerows and produces wonderful white blossom and red seeds.

Hops (Humulus lupulus), produces vine-like leaves and green, yellow scented flowers. It is cultivated throughout Europe.

Horse-radish (Cochlearia armoracia), is a wild plant which is also cultivated. It has long coarse leaves and white or pink flowers.

Hyssop (Hyssopus officinalis), grows around ruined buildings, including old monasteries. It has small blue-purple flowers.

Liquorice (Glycyrrhiza glabra), is a native plant of Southern Asia and Europe. It was cultivated by the Greeks, Persians and the Romans. The monks of England knew of its stomach ulcer-healing ability and its value as a laxative.

Liverwort (Anemone hepatica), this herb originates from temperate Northern zones. Its lobulated leaves were thought to resemble the structure of the liver. It should be noted that there is also an *English Liverwort* (Peltigera canina), which is actually a greyish lichen seen on old dykes and walls.

Lungwort (Sticta pulmonaria), also called *Oak Lungs and Lung Moss*, grows in woods and thickets. Its spotted leaves resemble lungs, hence the belief that it was useful in lung and respiratory problems.

Marsh Cudweed (Gnaphalium uliginosum) is a well known herb which when made into an infusion, makes an excellent remedy for dabbing on cold sores. It is a branched, stalked plant with elliptical leaves and crowded looking flowers. It is common throughout Europe.

Marshmallow (Althaea officinalis), is a tall plant found near the coast. It has soft, hairy leaves, and small pale-pink flowers.

Meadowsweet (Flipendula ulmaria), is a meadow or bankside herb with red stemmed, compound fern-like leaves and cream coloured flowers.

The Mints including Peppermint (Mentha piperita) are all distinguished by their odour and taste.

Mustard (Sinapsis alba), also called *Gold Dust,* is a commonly grown indoor herb.

Nettle (Urtica urens), the *Common Stinging Nettle,* also called *Sting-leaf* and *Bad Man's Plaything*. It has a long hard hairy stem with characteristic serrated leaves. The flowers can be surprisingly beautiful.

Nutmeg (Myristica fragans), was thought to be effective in all mental and brain disorders because of the resemblance of the nutmeg to the surface of the brain.

Parsley (Carum petroselinum), taken as in infusion also has a long history of usage for urinary gravel. It was used by the monks of Annaghadown. It is commonly cultivated in gardens and has typical curled foliage and a distinctive smell.

Parsley Piert (Alchemilla arvensis), also called *Breakstone* or *Colicwort*. It is a small wild flower found in sandy soils. The flowers are tiny and are just as green as the rest of the plant. It rarely grows more than three or four inches in height.

Periwinckle (Vinca major) has paired, glossy green leaves. It propagates itself by running stems, so that it will take over an area of soil, choking other plants.

Plantain (Plantago major), commonly grows on waste ground. It is also known as *Snakeweed, Englishman's foot and St. Patrick's Leaf*. Its long flat ribbed leaves were considered a sign that it could be used to treat ailments associated with the hands, feet, the fingers or the nerves.

Pleurisy Root (Asclepias tuberosa) comes from America where it prefers peaty soil. It grows to about two feet in height and has deep yellow or bright orange flowers.

Pumpkin (Cucurbita maxima), also called *Wormseed*. For centuries the seeds of the pumpkin have been used to expel worms from the body.

Rose (Rosacea), this comes in many forms, as all gardeners will know. Its characteristic leaves and flowers are recognisable around the world.

Sage (Salvia officinalis), grows to about three feet in height as a small bush herb. It has eliptical narrow leaves with purple flowers.

St John's Wort (Hypericum perforatum), also called *Holy Herb, Balm to the Warrior's Wound, Touch and Heal*. This herb in mediaeval times was thought to have been imbued with healing powers because it blooms around the time of the Saint's Day. The red juice of its curiously perforated leaves were thought to represent the blood of the saint and its ability to cure wounds.

Self-Heal, (Prunella vulgaris), also called *All Heal, Sicklewort and Hookweed*. It grows close to the ground and throws out distinctive violet coloured flowers which have a distinctive spike, like a hook or a sickle.

Skullcap (Scutellaria galericulata), also called *Hoodwort and Helmet Flower*. This is a very famous herb which has been used for centuries. The flowers shaped like a helmet with the visor closed was thought to indicate its value in disorders of the mind and the head.

Shepherd's Purse (Capsella bursa-pastoris), also called *Shepherd's Heart and Sanguinary*, grows on the sides of roads and waste ground. Its tiny seed boxes, like Shepherd's purses, or tiny hearts, imply its use in heart and circulatory problems.

Strawberry (Fragaria vesca), because of the resemblance of the fruit to the shape of the heart, it was perceived to be of value in heart disorders.

Thyme (Thymus vulgaris), grows to about a foot in height. it has masses of grey green leaves and purplish florets in Spring.

Valerian (Valeriana officinalis), also called *All Heal* (so do not confuse with Self-Heal), *St George's Herb* and *Garden Heliotrope*. It grows to about four feet in height and has toothed leaves and beautiful pale pink tubular florets.

Vervain (Verbena officinalis) grows to about three feet in height. It has broad basal toothed leaves and fine two-lipped lavendar like flowers.

Walnut (Juglans nigra), a tree which produces characteristic wrinkled nuts. The nut was thought to resemble the convoluted surface of the brain, hence the nuts were considered to be valuable in disorders of the mind and of the brain.

Willow (Salix alba), a tree that classically grows in damp places because it is a 'water-lover.' Its drooping, sad hanging appearance is quite characteristic.

Witch Hazel (Hamamelis virginiana), grows in woods and near water. It looks rather like comon hazel but the leaves are smaller and have distinct veins. It produces bright yellow spidery flowers.

Wormwood (Artemisia absinthium), also called *Green Ginger*. This is possibly the bitterest of all plants. It is a herb which should only be taken under the supervision of a doctor or herbalist.

Yarrow (Acillea millefolium), also called *Bloodwort*, *Woundwort* and *Staunch-weed*. This wild plant grows alongside country paths and lanes. It throws off great 'daisy-bunch' flowers.

Yellow dock (Rumex crispus), grows by roadsides and in ditches. It has six inch long leaves which are slightly curled at the edge.

Selected Bibliography

Although this book is very much about the oral tradition of Folk Medicine and has been based to a very large extent upon remedies which I have had *'passed onto me'* by word of mouth, it would be impossible to research such a subject without lots of guidelines. The following selected bibliography provided me with many of those guides.

BAKER, M. *Folklore and Customs of Rural England* London: David and Charles, 1988

BREWER. *The Dictionary of Phrase and Fable* Ware: Wordsworth, 1993

BUCHMAN,D. D. *Herbal Medicine* New York: Gramercy, 1989

CERES. *The Healing Power of Herbal Teas* Wellingborough, Thorsons, 1988

CHAUNDLER, C. *A Year Book of Customs* Oxford: Mowbray, 1957

CHAUNDLER, C. *A Year Book of Folk-Lore* Oxford: Mowbray, 1959

DE VRIES, J. *Traditional Home and Herbal Remedies* Edinburgh: Mainstream, 1987

DE BAIRACLI LEVY, J.*The Illustrated Herbal Handbook for Everyone* London: Faber and Faber, 1988

DOANE, N. L. *Indian Doctor Book* Charlotte, North Carolina: Aerial Photography Services, 1985

EBERTIN, R. *Astrological Healing* Wellingborough: Aquarian Press, 1990

FABREGA, H. *Disease and Social Behaviour* Cambridge, Massachusetts: MIT Press, 1974

FRAYLING, C. *The Face of Tutankhamun* London: Faber and Faber, 1992

GORDON, L. *A Country Herbal* Exeter: Webb and Bower, 1980

GRIEVE, M. *A Modern Herbal* London: Tiger, 1992

HELMAN, C,G. *Culture, Health and Illness* Bristol, Wright, 1990

HERNE, A *The Seaside Holiday* London: Cresset Press, 1967

JARVIS, D. C. *Folk Medicine* London: Pan,

JARVIS, D. C. *Arthritis and Folk Medicine* London: Pan, 1970

JONES, A. *Dictionary of Saints* Ware: Wordsworth, 1992

JOSEPH, H. *Shakespeare's Son-in-law: John Hall, Man and Physician* New York, 1993

KEYTE, G. *The Mystical Crystal* Saffron Walden: C.W.Daniel, 1993

KLEINMAN, A. *Patients and Healers in the Context of Culture* Berkeley: University of California Press, 1981

KOHN, R. and WHITE. K.L. *Health Care – An International Study* Oxford University Press, 1977

LYONS, A. S. and PETRUCELLI, R. J. *Medicine – An Illustrated History* New York: Abradale, 1987

McGREGOR-ROBERTSON, J. *The Household Physician* London: Gresham, circa 1910

McKEOWAN, T. *The Role of Medicine* Princeton: Princeton University Press, 1979

MILLS, S. Y. *The A–Z of Modern Herbalism* London: Thorsons, 1989

MILLS, S. Y. *The Essential Book of Modern Herbal Medicine* London: Penguin, 1991

NEUBERT, O. *Tutankhamun* London, Mayflower, 1972

OPIE, I. and TATEM, M. *A Dictionary of Superstitions*, Oxford University Press, 1992

OSLER, W. *The Practice of Medicine* New York: Appleton, 1910

PALMER, R. *Britain's Living Folklore* London: David and Charles, 1991

PELMER COSMAN, M. *Medieval Holidays and Festivals* London: Piatkus,1981

PETULENGRO, G. *Romany Remedies and Recipies* London: Methuen, 1935

QUERESHI, B. *Transcultural Medicine* Lancaster: Kluwer Academic, 1990

RINZLER, C. A. *Dictionary of Medical Folklore* Ware: Wordsworth, 1991

ROBINSON, M. *The New Family Herbal* London: Nicholson, circa 1914

ROOK, T. *Roman Baths in Britain* Princes Riseborough: Shire, 1992

SIGERIST, H. E. *History of Medicine* Oxford University Press, 1977

TEMKIN, O. *Galenism: Rise and Decline of a Medical Philosophy* Ithaca, New York: Cornell University Press, 1973

THOMAS, W. and PAVITT, K. *The Book of Talismans* London: Bracken Books, 1993

WALLIS BUDGE, E. A. *Egyptian Magic,* London: Paul, Trench, Trubner, 1899

WARD, J. *Dreams and Omens* London: Foulsham, circa 1965

WALVIN, J. *Beside the Seaside,* London: Allen Lane 1978

WHEELWRIGHT, E.G. *Medicinal Plants and their History*: New York: Dover, 1974

Useful Addresses

Britain

Astrology

THE ASTROLOGICAL
ASSOCIATION,
396 Caledonian Road,
London, N1 1DN

BRITISH ASTROLOGICAL AND
PSYCHIC SOCIETY,
124 Trefoil Crescent,
Broadfield,
Crawley,
West Sussex, RH11 9EZ

Bach Flower Remedies

BACH FLOWER REMEDIES Ltd,
Unit 6,
Suffolk Way,
Drayton Road,
Abingdon,
Oxon, OX14 5JX

THE Dr EDWARD BACH CENTRE,
Mount Vernon,
Sotwell,
Wallingford,
OXON, OX10 0PZ

Crystals

Crystal 2000,
37 Bromley Road,
St Annes-on-Sea,
Lancashire, FY8 1PQ

Dowsing

THE BRITISH SOCIETY OF
DOWSERS,
Sycamore Cottage,
Tamley Lane,
Hastingleigh,
Ashford,
Kent.

THE RADIONICS ASSOCIATION,
Baerlein House,
Goose Green,
Deddington,
Banbury,
OXON, OX15 0SZ

Folklore

THE FOLKLORE SOCIETY,
c/o University College,
Gower Street,
London, WC1E 6BT

Herbalism

NATIONAL INSTITUTE OF
MEDICAL HERBALISTS,
65 Frant Road,
Tunbridge Wells, Kent.

NEAL'S YARD APOTHECARY,
Neal's Yard,
Covent Garden,
London, WC2

POTTER'S HERBAL SUPPLIES Ltd,
Leyland Mill Lane,
Wigan,
Lancs, WN1 2SB

Homoeopathy

THE BRITISH HOMOEOPATHIC
ASSOCIATION,
27a Devonshire Street,
London, W1N 1RJ

THE FACULTY OF
HOMOEOPATHY,
The Royal London Homoeopathic
Hospital,
Great Ormond Street,
London, WC1N 3HR

THE UNITED KINGDOM
HOMOEOPATHIC MEDICAL
ASSOCIATION,
6 Livingstone Road,
Gravesend,
Kent, DA12 5DZ

THE SOCIETY OF
HOMOEOPATHS,
2 Artizan Road,
Northampton, NN1 4HU

THE HOMOEOPATHIC SOCIETY,
2 Powis Place,
Great Ormond Street,
London, WC1N 3HT

Hydrotherapy

THE ROYAL PUMP ROOM,
Leamington Spa,
Warks.

Naturopathy

BRITISH NATUROPATHIC AND
OSTEOPATHIC ASSOCIATION,
6 Netherall Gardens,
London, NW3 5RR

Abroad

Herbalism

USA
AMERICAN HERB ASSOCIATION,
Box 353, Rescue, CA 95672

AUSTRALIA
NATIONAL HERBALISTS
ASSOCIATION OF AUSTRALIA,
27 Leith Street, Coorparoo,
Queensland 4151

Homoeopathy

AFRICA
AFRICAN HOMOEOPATHIC
MEDICAL FEDERATION,
PO Box 131, Nempi, Oru L.G.A., Imo
State, Nigeria, Africa

INDIA
HAHNEMANNIAN SOCIETY OF
INDIA,
476 Gautam Nagar, New Delhi 110
949 India

NEW ZEALAND
NEW ZEALAND HOMOEOPATHIC
SOCIETY,
PO 2939, Auckland, New Zealand

SOUTH AFRICA
HOMOEOPATHIC SOCIETY OF
SOUTH AFRICA,
PO Box 9658, Johannesburg 2000,
South Africa

AUSTRALIA
AUSTRALIAN INSTITUTE OF
HOMOEOPATHY,
21 Bulah Close, Berowra Heights,
Sydney NSW 2082

FRANCE
LIGA MEDICORM
HOMOEOPATHIC
INTERNATIONALIS,
1068 21025 Dijon Cedex, France

DOLISOS, (Manufacturer)
62, rue Beaubourg 75003, Paris,
France

USA
AMERICAN FOUNDATION FOR
HOMEOPATHY,
1508 S Garfield, Alhambra, CA
91801, USA

HOMEOPATHIC EDUCATIONAL
SERVICES,
2124 Kittredge Street, Berkeley, CA
94704, USA

NATIONAL CENTER FOR
HOMEOPATHY,
801 N. Fairfax, Suite 306, Alexandria,
VA 22314

Natural Medicine

SRI LANKA,
MEDICINE ALTERNATIVE,
28 International Buddhist Centre
Road, Colombo 6

Index

The main entry for a condition (covering all five types of remedy where appropriate) and for a remedy is indicated by bold page numbers. Additional specific references have been included as subheadings.

for eye problems, 148, 156
for insomnia, 172
for jealousy, 173
for night terrors, 179
for styes, 190
emetics, 72
emperors, curative powers, 35–6
English Liverwort (*Peltigera canina*),
65, **209**
Englishman's Foot *see* Plantain
epilepsy, **154–5**
charms for, 35, 37
healing vessels, 42
magical cures, 26
patron saints, 32, 33
plant remedies, 41
Epsom baths, 96–7
Eros, 100
erysipelas 33 **155–6** *and see* shingles
Essences, 71–3
evil eye, 28–9
amulets against, 30–1, 35, 37, 39,
122
plant remedies, 41
evil influences, 37, 38
evil spirits, 62
exhaustion, 114
Eye of Horus, 30–1
eye problems, **156–7**
birth-stones, 37
healing vessels, 43, 64
and healing waters, 89
patron saints, 32
plant remedies, 41
stones for, 38, 155, 187
and see black eye; conjunctivitis;
styes
Eyebright (*Euphrasia officinalis*), **63–4,
208**
for eye problems, 148, 156, 190

F
face pack, 147
fainting, **157**
fasting, 25

fear, **157–8**, 164
feet, **158–9**
baths, 97, 130
herbal remedies, 79, 82
plant remedies, 66, 164
and see chilblains; corns
Fennel (*Foeniculum vulgara*), **208**
for arthritis, 135
for problems associated with cold, 80
for constipation, 148
for infertility, 171
for love, 106
for obesity, 180
fertility, 25, 30, 42, 80, 98–100 *and see*
conception charms; contraceptives
fever, 42, 61, 67, 77, **159**
Feverfew (*Chrysanthemum Parthenium*), **208**
for arthritis, 135
for problems associated with cold, 80
for headache, 165
for menstrual problems, 177
for nosebleeds, 180
Figwort (*Scrophularia nodosa*), 64, **208**
for problems associated with cold, 79
for eczema, 154
for haemorrhoids, 163
for injury, 171
for wounds, 196
fingers, 66, 181 *and see* hands
Fitzgerald, Dr William, 120
flatulence, **159–60**
Foxglove (*Digitalis purpurea*), 64, **208**
for oedema, 181
France, folk medicine, 17
freckles, **160**
frogs
for addiction, 131
for bed-wetting, 137–8
for coughs, 149
for hangovers, 164
for hoarseness, 168
for incontinence, 169
in love potions, 175
for mouth ulcers, 26, 178